Empowerment and the Health Service User

volume two

James Dooher and Richard Byrt

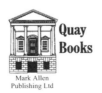
Quay
Books

Mark Allen
Publishing Ltd

Quay Books Division, Mark Allen Publishing Limited, Jesses Farm,
Snow Hill, Dinton, Wiltshire, SP3 5HN

British Library Cataloguing-in-Publication Data
A catalogue record is available for this book

© Mark Allen Publishing Ltd 2003
ISBN 1 85642 227 5

Printed in the UK by The Cromwell Press, Trowbridge, Wiltshire

**Empowerment and the
Health Service User**

Also published by Quay Books:

Empowerment and Participation: Power, influence and control in contemporary health care, volume one
edited by James Dooher and Richard Byrt

This book is dedicated to Fran Dooher, who empowered people and communities in Leicester.

Contents

List of contributors

Anonymous contributor is Irish and has had a historical diagnosis of paranoid schizophrenia. Following meaningful intervention by a far-sighted psychiatrist, he now deals with stress by utilising alternative treatments. He works in the voluntary sector, having occasional interludes of strategic involvement in mental health affairs.

Tony Booth works for a Midlands Social Services Department managing a team whose objective is to keep children and young people out of care.

Anthony Bree joined the staff of a Therapeutic Community in 1993 and has worked in the Outreach Team since it was set up in January 2000.

Caroline Byrt CQSA, DBA is an interim senior manager within social services settings, specialising in the modernisation of services and organisation change management, with an interest in service user and carer participation.

Richard Byrt RMN, RNLD, RGN, PhD Bsc (Hons) is Clinical/ Education Facilitator at Arnold Medium Secure Unit, Nottinghamshire Healthcare NHS Trust, and the School of Nursing and Midwifery, De Montfort University.

Penelope Campling is Consultant Psychotherapist at Francis Dixon Lodge therapeutic community in Leicester.

Martin Carter is Director of Communications for Somerset Health Authority. Soon after joining Somerset in 1995, his role was extended to encompass a lead role for the authority in promoting and developing user and public participation in the NHS.

James Dooher RMN, MA, FHE, Cert Ed, Dip HCR is Senior Lecturer and Pathway Leader for Mental Health at De Montfort University and Clinical Coach for Leicestershire and Rutland Healthcare Trust.

Jenny Fisher trained as a nurse at the Royal London Hospital. She has been actively involved with Rethink, formerly the National Schizophrenia Fellowship, for many years. She was elected to the

National Chair of Rethink in January 1999 and held this office until January 2003.

Paul Fitzgerald is a Sexuality Counsellor with North Warwickshire Primary Care Trust. He is a Relate trained remedial therapist and has recently qualified as a psychosexual therapist. He is a member of an External Reference Group who advise the Department of Health.

Jane Godfrey has worked as a nurse within mental health and as a senior lecturer at the University of the West of England. She has returned to practice in general medicine and is currently working as a staff nurse with the United Bristol Health Care Trust.

Jackie Green is Principal Lecturer in Health Promotion at Leeds Metropolitan University and Head of the Centre for Health Promotion Research and also Editor-in-Chief of *Promotion and Education*.

John Hyslop works as the Manager of Oxfordshire Mental Health Matters. He has spent four years conducting research with the National Schizophrenia Fellowship (now Rethink) and the Revolving Doors Agency.

Wendy Ifill is a young black woman who writes stories, poetry and articles for academic journals. She has used mental health services for twenty-two years.

Ann Jackson is Senior Practice Development Fellow with the RCN Institute Mental Health Programme.

Mark RD Johnson is Professor of Diversity in Health and Social Care at Mary Seacole Research Centre, De Montfort University, Leicester.

Susan Liderth became a patient on an acute mental health ward in Leicester five years ago.

Nessa McHugh is a Senior Midwifery Lecturer at De Montfort University. Her current research interest is in story telling, and the dissemination of midwifery knowledge.

Dr Nicky Pearson is Director of Clinical Governance for Somerset Health Authority.

Roger Phillips BA (Hons) is a broadcaster for BBC Radio Merseyside.

Bob Sang is widely regarded as one of the UK's leading independent practitioners in the participatory development of modern health systems: linking the engagement of patients and the public with the learning that sustains organisational, social and services innovation.

Rosemary Simpson is a Research and Development Officer for Leicestershire and Rutland Healthcare NHS Trust. Working within the Psychiatry for the Elderly Directorate, she has primary responsibility for leading the research agenda and ensuring an evidence base is translated into care.

Mahendra Solanki is a poet, lecturer and creative writing tutor. He teaches at Nottingham Trent University, where he leads the MA in writing programme.

'Sue' describes herself as a thirty-eight-year-old patient currently living in a rehabilitation unit which she feels is much better than acute care.

Keith Tones is Emeritus Professor of Health Promotion at Leeds Metropolitan University.

Marian Weeks is an orthopaedic pre-admissions sister at Nevill Hall Hospital, Gwent Health Care NHS Trust.

Andrew Wetherell is an Associate Consultant with the Sainsbury Centre for Mental Health and runs a freelance mental health training and development consultancy. He has worked in the UK Mental Health Service User Movement since early 1994 and his work has included developing self-help support initiatives and managing advocacy services.

Roberta Graley-Wetherell is a founding member and former National Co-ordinator of the United Kingdom Advocacy Network and Founder Chairperson of the European Network of Users and Ex-users in Mental Health. She runs a freelance mental health training and development consultancy.

Acknowledgements

Our thanks to:

Marjory Bancroft
Eileen Byrt
WH Byrt
Elizabeth Dooher
Millicent Dooher
Maeve Holmes
Sarah Honeychurch
Karen L Jackson

Chris Lomas
Norman Long
John McClelland
Jim McDonald
Paul Pleasance
Kath Sanders
Adrian Webb
Gerald Wistow

The editors would like to acknowledge, with thanks, the following for granting copyright permission to publish material from work previously published elsewhere:

❖ IBC UK Conferences Limited for copyright permission to publish material in *Chapters 15* and *16*, previously published in: IBC UK Conferences Limited (2000) *Involving Users in Clinical Governance. Working with Users to Provide a Quality Service. LH183. Conference Handbook for One Day Conference.* 31 March 2000 at The Marlborough Hotel, London.

All royalties from this publication will be donated to Rethink (previously The National Schizophrenia Fellowship) and Marie Curie Cancer Care.

Foreword

While Parsons' influential description of the 'sick role' as a state wherein the person experiencing ill health implies a loss of power, the condition of 'user' of health services does not require total disempowerment. Indeed, in a market-driven healthcare system, the purchaser may have considerable influence. This problematic might, however, be overcome by consideration of the concept of 'active patient-hood' discussed by Byrt and Dooher in the introductory chapter. Nevertheless, there does remain a sense in which the patient or 'user', to obtain help and undergo healing, must surrender some autonomy to the health professional charged with their care, as this is part of the process of recovering responsibility and acknowledging the illness (Mechanic, 1962). Equally, the role of the professional is important — as Balint notes, 'patients can more easily tolerate diagnosed (ie. labelled) than undiagnosed pain' (Balint, 1968: 263).

The situation is not quite the same in the case of the carer, or other possible stakeholders with an interest in the health of an end-user (also sometimes known as a patient) — but the research and policy literature has been slow to come to grips with the complexity of these roles or, indeed, to consider the 'non-user' and the involuntary user. All of these previously under-heard constituencies are represented in this collection — which gives weight to the providers of 'care', so that there is fairness all round: exclusion of the professional with their expert knowledge from debates can be as harmful as exclusion of the user with all their experience.

The collection of essays in this volume explores the issues around these contested roles. Some of the core concepts have been more deeply discussed in volume I (Dooher and Byrt, 2002), but it is clear that the question can be looked at from (at least) two or more perspectives: hopefully, readers will find that this collection complements the other, while not contradicting it. Some new arenas or dimensions of exclusion are introduced, such as issues around sexuality (*Chapter 6*, *Chapter 7*), alongside ways of overcoming or combating these problems. All the authors are concerned to illuminate the potential for raising the efficacy and quality of the healthcare process by greater involvement of the 'end-user' and to demonstrate the mutual nature of the transaction.

It is important in any transaction — or joint activity, such as healing or caring, to pay attention to the 'role' of all the actors in the situation. This includes both the patient and the clinical professional, and any carers, all of whom have a valid voice — as is shown by Simpson (*Chapter 9*), or in an innovative look at the 'therapeutic community' with the voices of psychiatrists, nurse and user (*Chapter 10*). The insights to be gained from reading Randle's diary (*Chapter 13*) are considerable, as are the stories of the Wetherells (*Chapter 17*), which should be required reading for anyone seeking to support (or start) a self-help group. Other new tools for self-reliance and empowerment include the arts (*Chapter 19*), radio (*Chapter 18*) or even (says an author!), writing (*Chapter 20*).

It may well be that despite personal feelings of inadequacy or hierarchy, the individual possesses more competence or power than they realise. Even the right to derogate from social responsibility, or act 'irresponsibly', may be a form of power that can be used. Similarly, the disruption caused to the health services by recent re-organisations have also provided some opportunities, as *Chapter 14* demonstrates. Equally, paying some attention to and reflection on one's own characteristics and behaviour may create a more effective or 'better' healer and carer.

As Balint considers that an essential for healing is the desire of the patient to 'want' to get better, the healer may be unable to heal without the active assistance or compliance of the sick person. This can only happen by 'active listening' to the would-be user. As Balint notes, 'If in doubt, do not hurry, but listen' (Balint, 1968: 275). The essays in this and its earlier sibling volume demonstrate the value of collaborative working, and the folly of attempting to force healing on the patient: certainly it is hard to 'make' someone better.

Mark RD Johnson
Professor of Diversity in Health and Social Care
Mary Seacole Research Centre
De Montfort University, Leicester
July 2002

References

Balint M (1968) *The Doctor, his Patient and the Illness*. Pitman Medical, London

Dooher J, Byrt R, eds (2002) *Empowerment and Participation: Power, influence and control in contemporary health care*. Quay Books, Mark Allen Publishing Limited, Salisbury, Wiltshire

Mechanic D (1962) The concept of illness behaviour. *J Chronic Dis* **15**: 189–94

Parsons T (1951) *The Social System*. The Free Press, Glencoe

1

'Service users' and 'carers' and their desire for empowerment and participation

Richard Byrt and James Dooher

As this book concerns service user and carer empowerment and participation, it seems appropriate to begin with a consideration of the question: who are service users and carers? Following definitions of empowerment and participation, the authors will consider types of participant as a dimension of participation; and the various stakeholders, including service users and carers, who are involved in health services. Terms used to describe service users and their roles in health services are outlined, with particular reference to consumerism. There follows a consideration of literature on carers and of stages of participation; and a review of some of the research on patients' and clients' wishes to participate and to be empowered. Some of the topics covered are considered in more depth in *Chapter 2*.

We have used the terms 'service user' and 'carer' only for reasons of clarity, as these terms are widely used in the literature and in Department of Health (DoH) documents. As will be noted later in this chapter, these terms are not acceptable to all people, eg. individuals who receive treatment against their will (Barnes and Bowl, 2001) and some people seen by professionals as providing care for relatives, partners or friends (Rogers, 2000). However, it is difficult to find alternative terms which would be universally acceptable.

Types of participant

Chapter 2 in the companion volume to this book explores the meaning and dimensions of empowerment and participation (Byrt and Dooher, 2002). The following definitions of these concepts are proposed, based on the research-based and other literature explored in that chapter.

Empowerment involves increases or transfers in power involving four dimensions. These include individual or psychological empowerment, in which the individual experiences increased power or control.

Other dimensions relate to service-initiated empowerment, where professionals or managers enable service users or carers to increase their power. Empowerment also includes the achievement of actual change (in health services and/or wider society); and social inclusion. Achieving the latter involves gaining greater power within society, with the availability of increased life opportunities, and the reduction of discrimination.

Participation is: … 'the involvement of service users/carers in responsibility and/or decision making, which has an intended impact on services and/or policies which affect the individual participant and/or other service users/carers…' (Byrt and Dooher, 2002, based on Byrt, 1994, p. 29). Participation can occur at different levels (from individual care to central government or global issues); and various degrees (from information/consultation to complete responsibility). Other dimensions of participation include its components or features; modes of influencing people in positions of power; and types of participant. Participation varies in the extent that it is formal or informal; explicitly related to individuals' experiences as service users/carers; and seen as an end in itself or as a means to achieve concrete goals (Byrt and Dooher, 2002).

Byrt and Dooher (2002) consider several dimensions included in typologies of participation. Many typologies do not include types of participant. Windle and Cibulka (1981) included a participant dimension in their multi-dimensional typology and classified participants in community mental health centres into 'communities', 'citizens', 'employees' and 'consumers'. Brager *et al* (1987) referred to four categories of participants in community groups, with varying amounts of involvement and commitment. In considering 'user involvement', a College of Health document comments:

> *… For the purpose of this document, the term user and carer are used to include patients, carers and patients' representatives, as well as the local community and wider public as potential patients and taxpayers…*

> (Kelson 1997, p. 2)

Williamson (1995) differentiated between 'patients and carers', 'consumer groups' and 'consumerists'. The last group include service users with an understanding of a wide range of interests and issues of concern to other clients/patients (Hogg, 1999, p. 100, citing Williamson, 1995). Braye (2000) refers to the need for members of wider communities to be participants in decisions about services; and argues that individuals should do so as 'citizens', rather than be marginalised in narrow roles as 'services users'. The term 'lay participation' has been used to refer to the involvement of members of the public, eg. in relation to primary care groups (Anderson, 2001). Bracht *et al* (1999) refer to the importance of identifying various participants, particularly, 'key leaders or influential patients or groups' (p. 92) for involvement in community organisations for health promotion. Wright (1999) offers a 'user involvement framework', produced for an NHS trust, which incorporates a check-list for 'who to involve in what', including service users/carers, 'groups of people sharing a particular service', 'communities of interest', and the 'general public' (Wright, 1999, p. 58f). A checklist produced by Priestley *et al* includes the participation of 'disabled people's organisations as well as individual users' (Priestley, 1999, p. 164, citing Gibbs and Priestley, 1995 and Priestley, 1996). The importance of ensuring that specific members of communities are involved has been stressed, eg. in relation to people from minority ethnic groups, women, individuals with disabilities, older people and carers (Barnes and Bowl, 2001; Chevannes, 2002; Patel and Fatimilehin, 1999; Barnes and Warren, 1999) (see also *Chapters 3* to *9).*

Other stakeholders in health services

The literature on types of participant reflects the large numbers of health service stakeholders, beside service users and carers (*Figure 1.1, p. 6*). The term 'stakeholder' is used here to refer to '…interested parties, each with rights and duties appropriate to their interest…' (Handy 1993, p. 388).

Brooks (2001) refers to the importance, in facilitating service user participation, of understanding the opposing priorities and discourses of clients/patients and other stakeholders. The latter, in their attempts to influence health services, often yield greater power than service users and carers, and the statutory bodies, voluntary organisations, and other bodies representing their interests (Hogg, 1999). Many of these stakeholders can be seen as 'service users' in some senses. They include taxpayers and other members of the public, almost all of whom will be clients/patients and/or involved as carers at various times in their lives (Hogg, 1999). Other stakeholders include; local and central government politicians, including ministers for health and their civil servants; various media (see *Chapter 18*); and managers of independent health services, and of the NHS at national, district health authority and trust level, including non-executive board members. Health authority and other purchasers of services are also 'service users'. When contracts for the supply of health services are relatively formal:

> *... the interests served in contracting are those of managers and politicians, who benefit from greater control of expenditure and activity and a more efficient service. However, if other organisational objectives, for example, quality or responsiveness to patients, are considered, the contracts are less explicit...*

> (Spurgeon *et al*, 1997, p. 149)

Health service professionals and other workers also seek to exert influence individually, and through their professional associations, trade unions and regulatory bodies such as the Nursing and Midwifery Council (NMC) and British Medical Association (Cameron, 1999). The particular power of medical staff has been outlined in relation to various areas of care (Miers, 1999; Saks, 2002). Godsell (1999) comments on the relative power of service users with learning disabilities and their carers versus professionals and managers:

> *... a set of ideas and values... have dominated the decision making processes that underlie policy and regulation. These ideas are embedded in the collected voices of the professionals — the doctors, managers, administrators and nurses... Their voices have overpowered the disparate voices of parents, carers and the users of the services. Their ability to create and control policy and provision indicates their capacity to wield power...*

> (Godsell, 1999, p. 207)

These comments refer to organisations in which the roles of 'service user', 'professional' and 'purchaser of services' are seen as distinct and separate. However, organisations run by and for 'service users' have been described (Chamberlin, 1988; Priestley 1997). Participants in these organisations do not have rigid or unchanging roles such as 'user', 'provider' and 'professional'. An example is an information desk run by Derbyshire Centre for Integrated Living, which '... suggests a blurring of the established hierarchy between "providers" and "users". In so doing, it illustrates how user participation can create opportunities for resistance to the discourse of "carers" and "cared for"'(Priestley, 1999, p. 197).

Some health services are influenced by specific stakeholders. For secure hospitals and units, these include the judiciary, the Home Office and local members of the public, politicians and media (Byrt, 2001), who may, for instance, campaign, opposing the service (see *Chapter 18*). In some services (eg. many nursing homes for older people) the main stakeholder is the individual or company owning it financially. Indeed, it has been argued that stakeholders with the greatest power are those with commercial interests. These include large, often global or multi-national financial organisations and pharmaceutical companies, which have considerable influence on which types of treatment are seen as appropriate (Hogg, 1999; Prior, 1999). Powerful political and commercial interests influence mothers' decisions about breastfeeding (Hogg, 1999); and dictate decisions about the distribution of medical supplies and other necessities for health in poorer countries (Stein, 1997).

Service user and carer participation and empowerment are influenced by the relative amounts of power held by these stakeholders; and the extent that the latter are prepared to share this (Lupton *et al*, 1998). Power may be shared in ways that reinforce the current dominant position or discourse, eg. in relation to beliefs of people in positions of power about what count as 'appropriate' treatments or 'healthy' or valued lifestyles or relationships (Miers, 1999). This point is considered by some of the contributors to this book and its companion volume. See, for example, *Chapters 6* and *9*, and Saks (2002). In relation to sharing power, some self-help groups and other voluntary organisations have been happy to receive pharmaceutical company funding. However, other bodies, such as Health Action International, have argued that this '… compromises… the right to receive independent and objective information…' (Hogg, 1999, p. 142). In some cases, commercial and political interests seriously constrain choice for particular service users, and the service provided. This is particularly the case with groups of individuals who lack power and who are marginalised in society. Examples include many older people who have been forced to contribute their savings and pensions towards nursing home care (Hogg, 1999). In secure units and hospitals, decisions about levels of security and restrictions of patients sometimes appear to be made, at least in part, for political reasons, eg. in response to adverse media publicity (Byrt, 2000; UKCC, 1999).

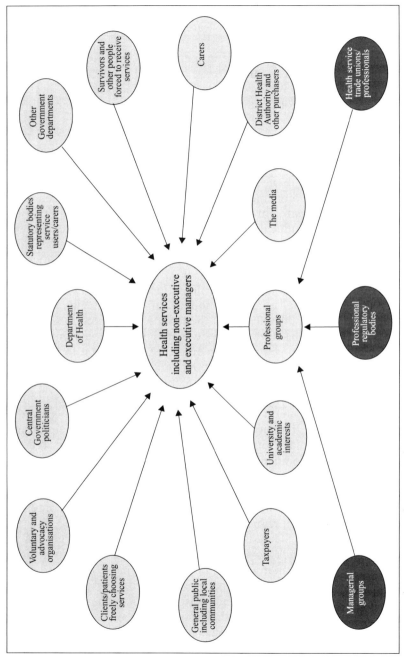

Figure 1.1: 'Service users', 'carers' and other stakeholders in health services

'Health service user' and other terms

The use of particular terms to describe health service users reflects their status, and in some cases, their actual or intended participation or empowerment. Prior to the twentieth century, terms such as 'beneficiary' and 'supplicant' denoted the recipient's passive and inferior role (Smith, 1987). The term 'patient' has been said to suggest passivity and/or acceptance of suffering (Brandon, 1981; Brooks and Gillam, 2001). '...The relative neglect of attempts to seek their views and understand their perceptions of health care may be the result of an image of older people as passive recipients of services...' (Littlechild and Glasby, 2000, p. 156). However, some authors note that recently, many service users are less prepared to accept care and treatment without question. This is said to be related to a rise in consumerism (see *Chapter 2*); and an increased awareness of service users' rights (Evans and Byrt, 2002; Hogg, 1999; Taylor, 1999). In particular, many recipients of learning disability and mental health services have challenged both professional expectations about patient/client roles and the care and treatment they have received. For several decades, a number of authors have associated the term 'psychiatric patient' with disempowerment, a failure by professionals to treat the individual as a whole person, and to see him/her only as someone who is 'mentally ill' (Barker, 1999; Barnes and Bowl, 2001; Chamberlin, 2000; Porter, 1991). In the UK, disempowering professional attitudes and treatment have been increasingly challenged since a growth, from the mid-1980s, of advocacy groups for individuals with learning disabilities (Walmsley and Downer, 1997) and of mental health survivors' movements (Barnes and Bowl, 2001; *Chapter 2*).

Terms coined by professionals or the public to denote (and sometimes stigmatise) certain groups of health service users have recently been challenged by many pressure groups (Oliver and Barnes, 1998; Sayce, 2000). For example, it has been argued that the typology and definitions of the International Classification of Impairment, Disability and Handicap (ICIDH) are based on assumptions that:

> *... people with impairments [should] be treated, changed, improved and made 'normal'... [The classification reflects] a particularly narrow set of Eurocentric values — namely, those of predominantly male, wealthy, middle class professionals... The work done on definitions has been*

> *carried out by people who do not themselves experience the daily problems of living and disability...*

(Oliver and Barnes, 1998, p. 15f)

Both Oliver and Barnes (1998) and Sayce (2000) refer to many health service users' definitions and meanings which '...have rejected the implications of the medical model of disability... [with] an explicit denial of a.... "disabled identity"...' (Oliver and Barnes, 1998, p. 18). The term 'service user' or 'user' has been rejected by some people because it does not reflect their own choice to use imposed mental health services or because of its connotations with drug use (Barnes and Bowl, 2001). Another word, often imposed, is 'victim':

> *... In my English class, I was pleased that 'My Left Foot' was included, but the booklet introduced Christy Brown's piece with 'Christy Brown was born a victim of cerebral palsy.' Now I have cerebral palsy. I have often been the victim of other people's attitudes, but I have never... felt myself to be a victim of cerebral palsy. When my English teacher found how I felt about the word victim, the whole class had a discussion about it. That was good for the thirty teenagers in my class, but what about the other 1400 in my school — especially those who've called me a freak, invalid, retarded and other fantastic words...*

(Corker and Davis, 2000, p. 228, quoting
Katy Caryer, 1999, 'a member of the disabled
children's group, "Young and Powerful"')

The above comments vividly illustrate some of the pejorative and stigmatising words still widely used to describe those of us who are living with physical disabilities, mental health problems and learning disabilities (Sayce, 2000). Participants in East Hertfordshire People First, a self-help group, have established a project to enable people with learning disabilities to respond effectively to verbal abuse. The organisation has also launched a campaign to raise awareness of the problem among the public, including schoolchildren (Salman, 2002). MIND found evidence of widespread discrimination and stigmatisation towards people with mental health problems (Barnes and Bowls, 2001). In one campaign, MIND questioned the use of stigmatising words:

> *Psycho?... People with mental health problems are more*
> *likely to be attacked than they are to attack others... Why*
> *use labels when they don't fit?*

(MIND, undated)

Certain words have been intentionally coined by professionals and managers to reflect changes which they have tried to effect in their relationships with service users. From the late 1940s, the word 'resident' was used to describe members of therapeutic communities who were receiving treatment. 'Resident' is considered to reflect more accurately the individual's involvement in decision making and responsibility in a democratic, permissive environment (Kennard, 1998; *Chapter 10*).

More recently, the term 'active patienthood' has been used to refer to some professionals' facilitation of health service users' active participation and the development of individual self-efficacy (Sturt, 1998). (Self-efficacy refers to an individual's belief that he/she is able to achieve specific goals [Tones and Green, 2002]). The term 'client' has reflected the wish of social workers and some health professionals to give individuals the rights and status of users of professional services (Smith, 1987). However, unlike the clients of most professionals, some people who receive health and social services do so reluctantly (Allen *et al*, 1992). In some cases, 'services' are imposed against people's will, as with mental health patients who are formally admitted, or people required to undergo compulsory HIV testing (Tannsjo, 1999). It has been argued that some health professionals, eg. those who work in secure hospitals and prisons, serve the interests of people other than, or in addition to, those of the client (Mason and Mercer, 1998).

In contrast to professional definitions, many recipients of health services, particularly those concerned with mental health, describe themselves as 'survivors' in order, '... to portray a positive image of people in distress and people whose experience differs from, or who dissent from, society's norms...' (Barnes and Bowl, 2001, p. 2, quoting http://www.inc.co.uk/-acorn/survivor.htm). Wallcraft and Michaelson (2001) refer to the need to develop, '... survivor discourse to replace the "psychopathology" of breakdown and crisis...' (Wallcraft and Michaelson, 2001, p. 177). There are many survivors' accounts which challenge the (often serious) oppression, stigmatisation and denial of basic rights which they have experienced (Chamberlin, 1988; Newnes *et al*, 2001; Sayce, 2000; Survivors' Poetry, Scotland 1996). Some of the contributors to this book outline such experiences (*Chapters 8, 12, 14* and *17*). The UK Survivors' Movement has grown considerably since the mid-1980s, with the development of several organisations, most notably, Survivors Speak Out and the UK Advocacy Network (UKAN) (Barnes and Bowl, 2001; *Chapter 2*).

'Carers'

The authors of this chapter are hesitant to use the term 'carers', as it is not a term used by some people so described. However, it will be used here for the sake of clarity, in view of its widespread use in the literature.

Rogers (2000) commented on the difficulty of defining 'carer'. Heron (1998) referred to, 'lack of clarity' and a 'number of levels of meaning' in the term. Several definitions refer to the notion of an unpaid individual (usually a relative, partner or friend) providing care, generally in the home of the person receiving the care (Carers National Association, 1998; Clayton, 1998; Ellis-Hill and Payne, 2001). For example, the foreword to a research study commissioned by The Princess Royal Trust for Carers included the following definition:

> ... *A carer is anybody who is helping to look after a partner, relative or friend who, because of illness, old age or disability, may not be able to manage at home without help... This resource of unpaid, committed partners, friends and relatives is truly at the heart of community care ...*

> (Butler, 1998, p. 2)

The term 'informal carer' is sometimes used to distinguish unpaid care from professional care. Some social care and health workers, particularly those who are untrained, are sometimes referred to as 'carers' (Heron, 1998; Webb and Tossell, 1999).

The term 'carer' became frequently used in the 1970s, in statutory services (Rogers, 2000) and, '... ideas about its role were developed largely from a professional perspective...' (Ellis-Hill and Payne, 2001, p. 156). The Carers (Recognition and Services) Act, 1995 defined a carer as a person who, '... provides or intends to provide a substantial amount of care on a regular basis...' (DoH, 1996a, p. 1). Earlier legislation recognised the existence of 'carers'. The Local

Government Act (1972) and the NHS Act (1977) enabled, but did not require, statutory services to provide support for carers. The Disabled Persons (Services, Consultation and Representation) Act, 1986 made it mandatory for local authority assessments to consider whether carers were able to give support, but did not consider their own needs. However, the NHS and Community Care Act (1990) required 'community care assessments' to consider carers' needs (Heron, 1998, p. 15, citing the above legislation). Despite official recognition in the Carers (Recognition and Services) Act, 1995, research has found that carers' needs are often inadequately assessed and met, with the perspectives of service users, rather than those of carers, influencing professional thinking (Nolan, 2001; citing Heaton *et al*, 1999 and other studies).

Many individuals involved in informal care do not see themselves as 'carers', and/or dislike the term (Heron, 1998). The latter has been criticised for failing to appreciate the reciprocity, or the complexity of relationships, in which people give and receive in a variety of mutually supporting ways (Bucknall and Holmes, 2001; DoH, 2001a; Nolan, 2001; Rogers, 2000). Indeed, individuals' lives and roles can be constrained if they are seen only as 'carers' or people 'in need of care', which can be the case, particularly for older people (*Chapter 9*) and individuals with learning disabilities (Barnes, 1997):

> *... Godfrey and Wistow... found that professionals tended not to demonstrate awareness of the fluidity and complexity of the carer/cared–for relationship...*
>
> (Preston-Shoot, 2000, p. 284, citing Godfrey and Wistow, 1997)

In Rogers' research, people described as 'carers':

> *... regard what they do as an extension of family or personal relations... Conceptually, the term ['carer'] centres on the performance of tasks which are both supportive in nature and grounded in pre-existing relationships of kinship or friendship... At what point does a partner, son, daughter or neighbour cease being such in order formally to take on the role of carer?...*
>
> (Rogers 2000, p. 113, citing Thomas, 1993)

Despite these reservations, the use of the term 'carer' has been said to enable people thus described to identify with others in similar situations; and to raise their visibility amongst the public, attracting charitable and business funding. Increased political visibility and power may also lead to health and social services policies that meet carers' needs (Heron, 1998). The Office of Population and Census Surveys estimated that in 1991, 'there were 6.8 million people defined as carers', 57% of whom were women (Payne and Ellis-Hill, 2001, p. 6).

Part of the literature has been criticised for assuming that 'carers' are a homogeneous group with similar needs (Barnes, 1997; Bucknall and Holmes, 2001; Rogers, 2000). Some research has not recognised the diversity of people so described, with the needs of, for example, black and very young carers remaining unrecognised (Dearden and Becker, 2000; Preston-Shoot, 2000). While family members constitute 90% of carers (Bucknall and Holmes, 2001, p. 127, citing HM Government, 1999), a significant proportion are friends or partners, including lesbians and gay men. Heaphy *et al* (1999) refer to 'non-heterosexual family formations', with partners, friends and blood relatives uniting to care for individuals living with AIDS. Sadly, the importance of partners or friends as the carers of lesbians and gay men has not always been recognised by health professionals (Godfrey, 1999; Wiltjon, 2000, citing the Royal College of Nursing, 1998; *Chapter 6*). The novel *Mates* includes a vivid and sad account of a health worker's failure to offer support to a gay man, or to recognise his loss after the death in hospital of his partner of thirty years (Wakefield, 1983).

It is often assumed that the needs and relationships of health service users and their carers will be sources of conflict (Barnes and Bowl, 2001), as in situations where an older individual wishes to return home from hospital, while his/her family consider that he/she needs admission to a nursing home (Teasdale, 1998). However, Barnes (1997) found from her research that such conflict was not inevitable, and that individuals with learning disabilities both contributed to their families, and were sometimes empowered by them. Nevertheless, McFadyen and Farrington (1997) recommended that, because carers' views are often ignored, '... user and carer issues should not be confused. Carer views need to be separated from user views and methodologies applied accordingly...' (McFadyen and Farrington, 1997, p. 264).

The literature refers to the importance of professionals recognising that carers have dual roles as experts/partners in care and as individuals with their own needs. Payne and Ellis-Hill (2001) refer to the typology of models of carers' roles formulated by Twigg and

Atkin (1994), with an addition by Nolan *et al* (1995). This typology includes 'carers as resources', where professionals assume that relatives will be able to provide care. Carers can also be seen as co-workers with professionals; or as co-clients, with their own needs. In 'superseded care', either the carer or the person receiving care decides that this should be discontinued, as in the case of young adults with disabilities who decide to live independently. Finally, Nolan *et al* (1995) suggested that 'the carer as expert' is an important role, with professional recognition of his/her experience and knowledge (Payne and Ellis-Hill, 2001, p. 8f).

However, a considerable amount of literature (some of it referred to in *Chapter 14* and in Evans and Byrt, 2002) refers to professionals ignoring carers, and failing to consult or otherwise communicate with them or recognise their expertise (Bucknall and Holmes, 2001; Gibson, 1995; Royal College of Physicians and College of Health, 1998; *Chapter 12*). Banks (2001) refers to central government policy (eg. *Caring about Carers*, HM Government, 1999) to increase the involvement of carers as partners in care with professionals. This is also emphasised in the *NHS Plan* (DoH, 2000b) and subsequent DoH requirements for the provision of staff education and training in this area (DoH, 2002). Some studies have found that many carers would like more information and greater participation in decisions concerning their loved ones when they are admitted to hospital. However, often carers are concerned about being seen to challenge or question staff in situations where the latter may hold more power in relation to what is seen as 'expert knowledge' and the control of information (May *et al*, 2001; Simons *et al*, 2001; Walker and Dewar, 2001). Furthermore, '... staff may characterise carers as "patients" when challenged by them...'; for example, assuming that their expressed concerns reflect guilt or personal failings (Walker and Dewar, 2001, p. 334, citing Allen, 2000).

The role of carers as partners in care may conflict with the meeting of their own needs.

> *...Carers may be seen simply as a resource to help hard-pressed staff to carry out their responsibilities, rather than as individuals with needs of their own...*

(Banks, 2001, p. 107)

One problem with the term 'carer' is that people may be seen only as 'carers', with a lack of appreciation of their other roles: '... Caregivers must be considered people first and consideration given to their full identity and multiple role...' (DoH, 2001a, quoting IASSID and WHO, 2000).

Research has demonstrated overwhelming needs in some carers, which are often unmet, and in the case of some individuals (eg. children and young people caring for parents) unrecognised (Dearden and Becker, 2000). Problems facing carers of specific minority ethnic groups have been highlighted (Chiu and Yu, 2001; Heron, 1998), including professionals' assumptions and stereotypes, for example, that all 'Asian carers are well supported by their extended families' (Heron, 1998, p. 79). Professionals sometimes fail to recognise that for many service users who are lesbian or gay, their partner is the most significant person, and often their main carer, who is also in need of support (Godfrey, 1999). Some carers, particularly those who are elderly, may be service users, in the sense of having as many or more health needs as the person they are caring for (Hogg, 1999; Rogers, 2000). The needs of carers of individuals with mental health problems are often unmet, and professionals have sometimes induced guilt feelings in parents of young people with schizophrenia (Bucknall and Holmes, 2001; *Chapter 12*). A carer of a partner diagnosed as having 'personality disorder' has described lack of professional support and information (Deborah, 1999). The need for support of relatives and partners of people who are dying, and the unmet needs of these carers have been highlighted (Andershed and Ternestedt, 2001; Taylor, 1999; DoH, 2000a). However, the NHS Cancer Plan (DoH, 2000a) emphasises the need for carers to receive support. *Chapter 13* outlines ways that carers' needs were met effectively in one hospital.

Professional — service user/carer relationships

Many survivors, including contributors to this book, describe disempowering and demeaning relationships and communication with professionals. (See Butler, 2002, for a poem by Susan Watters vividly describing authoritarian attitudes in a mental health nurse.) Some aspects of service user and carer empowerment and participation are particularly influenced by professional-service user/ carer relationships. Several authors (including some contributors to this book and its companion volume, Dooher and Byrt, 2002) have examined participation and empowerment specifically at the individual level within these relationships (Saks, 2002). Hogg refers to, '... changing and often contradictory expectations that underlie the rights and responsibilities of patients and professionals...' (Hogg, 1999, p. 5); and mentions four models which influence the relationship between health service users and professionals:

Paternalism:	*Professionals are deemed to know best and patients are required to trust them...'*
Consumerism:	*... Individuals are in charge of getting the best buy for their own health care and they cannot take the trustworthiness of professionals for granted...*
Autonomy:	*... puts respect for the individual first and recognises the different perspectives of patients and professionals...*
Partnership:	*... sees the giving and receiving of health care as a negotiation agreed between the parties...*

(Hogg, 1999, p.5)

Related to partnership models of professional-service user/carer relationships, are the notions of 'expert patients' and 'expert carers', who have becomes authorities on the health needs, care and treatment of themselves or loved ones, particularly in relation to long-standing illnesses and disabilities (Florin and Coulter, 2001; Kohner and Hill, 2000; Payne and Ellis-Hill, 2001). The idea of the 'patient as expert' is founded on '... the conviction that only a person who is experiencing a specific condition really knows what it is like...' (Florin and Coulter, p. 49). However, research suggests that service users' views are sometimes dismissed, with decisions made mostly by professionals (Miers, 1999; Paterson, 2001).

'The Degner Scale' (Degner and Sloan, 1992, cited in Robinson and Thomson, 2001) was produced to ascertain service users' preferences for roles in medical decision making (*Box 1.1*).

The notion that the service user or carer, like the customer, 'knows best' in relation to decisions about his/her treatment is one of the tenets of consumerism, which will be considered next.

> ❖ 'I prefer to make the final selection about which treatment I receive.
> ❖ I prefer to make the final selection of my treatment after seriously considering my doctor's opinion.
> ❖ I prefer that my doctor and I share responsibility for deciding which treatment is best for me.
> ❖ I prefer that my doctor makes the final decision about which treatment will be used, but seriously considers my opinion.
> ❖ I prefer to leave all decisions regarding my treatment to my doctor.'

Box 1.1: Degner's scale of decision-making preferences (Degner and Sloan, 1992, quoted in Robinson and Thomson, 2001)

Service users and carers as 'consumers'

According to Hogg:

> ... *Consumerism sees the individual as a client in the market place. The client looks for the best deal... Being a client also requires having choice...*

> (Hogg 1999, p. 48)

Lupton *et al* (1998, p. 50) point out that consumerism in economics is concerned with individuals' '... need for information, access, choice and redress in relation to specific services/products...'. The relationship between doctor/nurse and patient has been influenced by the latter's social class and wealth. Wealthy people have usually been consumers, in the economic sense, of private medical and nursing services. These 'consumers' have included both people receiving treatment and their carers, depending on who paid for the service. Klein pointed out that until 1911, when National Insurance was introduced, most doctors had limited salaries and social status (Klein, 1973). In relation to working class people, general practitioners were:

> ... *in the position of small tradesmen who had to do as instructed by the **customer**... [especially] practitioners who were engaged in...'contract medicine'... whereby doctors were hired by Friendly Societies... and similar associations to look after their members...*

> ... *In the circumstances of working-class general practice at the turn of the [nineteenth] century... the **customer** was always right, but... insisted on cheap medicine...*

> (Klein, 1973, p. 62f. Present authors' emphasis)

From the days of the Friendly Societies, service users have had some choice in deciding their general practitioners. During negotiations concerned with the National Insurance Act, 1911, the British Medical Association stressed that, 'free choice of doctor by patient' was essential (Klein, 1973, p. 64). Under the National Insurance Act, patients could choose any general practitioner from panels selected by Insurance Committees. Choice of hospital treatment depended on ability to pay, and was usually limited for poorer people using the voluntary hospital system before World War II, or for National Health Service patients (Klein, 1973). The following comments are still relevant today, and apply to carers choosing a service with, or on behalf of, relatives or partners, as well as service users:

> *... To talk about someone as a consumer normally implies he has freedom of choice... [and] has the information required to exercise that choice rationally... The consumer of medical services is very rarely in such a happy position... the more he needs medical services (ie. the more acutely ill he is), the less choice he has...*

(Klein, 1973, p. 157)

From the 1950s, recipients of private medicine were often referred to as 'consumers', particularly in American literature. During the 1970s, British NHS patients were increasingly described by this term, especially in papers on patient satisfaction. This decade saw an increased interest in what were often referred to as 'consumer views', which was reflected in the setting up in 1969 of the Hospital (later Health) Advisory Service, to assess health services for older people and patients with learning disabilities and mental health problems, following a series of scandals in long-stay hospitals (Jones, 1993; Martin with Evans, 1984). Several studies of clients' views were conducted, including a survey by the Royal Commission on the NHS, of patients' attitudes to their treatment (Royal Commission on the NHS, 1979).

From the early seventies, several Department of Health and Social Services (DHSS)/Department of Health publications referred to the importance of considering the needs and views of 'consumers'. Under Conservative governments between 1979 and 1997, there was increased emphasis on consumerism. The concept was endorsed in the NHS Management Enquiry Report (the Griffiths Report, DHSS, 1983) which emphasised evaluating quality in health services (Ham, 1985, p. 1), particularly from the viewpoint of the patient, who is often referred to in the report as the 'consumer' or 'customer'. There were several references to patients, and account was taken of, '... the interests of the patient, the community, the taxpayer and the employees...' (DHSS, 1983, p. 11). However, there were no references to the carer as 'consumer'. In the report, close parallels were drawn between health services and the commercial market. It was recommended that Health Authorities should assess service users' views through market research and other means (DHSS, 1983, p. 9).

> *... Businessmen have a keen sense of how well they are looking after their customers. Whether the NHS is meeting the needs of the patient, and the community, and can prove that it is doing so, is open to question...*
>
> (Ham, 1985, p. 1, quoting DHSS, 1983, p. 10)

The report further recommended:

> *... The Management Board and Chairmen should ensure that it is central to the approach of management, in planning and delivering services for the population as a whole, to:*
> *1. ascertain how well the service is being delivered at local level by obtaining the experience and perceptions of patients and the community...*
> *2. respond directly to this information;*
> *3. act on it in formulating policy;*
> *4. monitor performance against it...*
>
> (DHSS, 1983, p. 9)

The Griffiths Report commented on health service management's lack of commitment to consumers of health services; and recommended the appointment of general managers to improve customer relations and to increase responsiveness to public and consumer expectations. Griffiths also recommended that ministers should review the National Health Service to ensure that this objective was being met (DHSS, 1983). The Griffiths Report appears to have influenced an increase in attempts to assess service users' satisfaction with health services and to be more responsive to their needs. By 1985, '... a National Association of Health Authorities survey found at least eighty schemes for improving responsiveness to the needs of its consumers...' (Hunt and Reynolds, 1985, p. 7).

Since the mid-1980s, many measures of health service users' and carers' views have been devised, in order to improve quality. Between 1991 and 1997, Patients' Charters stressed the rights of patients, the standards of service they could expect and the value attached to patients' views (DoH, 1991; DoH, 1996b; DoH, 1997b). The monitoring of services and the meeting of service users' and carers' needs have been stressed in several DoH documents, including the White Paper *The new NHS — modern, dependable* (DoH, 1997a); *A First Class Service: Quality in the New NHS* (DoH, 1998); in National Service Frameworks (DoH, 1999; DoH, 2001b) and the *NHS Plan* (DoH, 2000b). These and other developments, in relation to central government policy since 1979, are considered in more detail in the next chapter.

Criticisms of consumerism

Critics have argued that most service users and carers are able to act as market consumers of health services only to a limited extent for several reasons. These and other criticisms of consumerism include the following:

❖ Most importantly, some clients, patients and carers, as well as certain professionals, object to the term 'consumer' because of its connotations with market ideologies with which they disagree (Barnes and Bowl, 2001).

❖ Even if the term is seen as appropriate, there are problems in defining 'who the consumer is' (Hogg, 1999, p. 169). This may include, for example, the health service user, carer, taxpayer, Health Authority or other purchaser of care, and other stakeholders (Hogg, 1999).

❖ It has been argued that consumerism does nothing to address wider imbalances of power (Barnes and Bowl, 2001; Priestley, 1999, citing Ramon, 1991 and Ritchie, 1994).

❖ Because of limited finances, most service users and carers have little choice but to use those NHS services that are provided (Hogg, 1999).

❖ NHS facilities sometimes offer limited choice, which for some services, vary in quality and availability in different parts of the country (Hogg, 1999). Some services are rationed (Hogg, 1999;

Lilley, 2000) or limited, eg. community services for older people discharged from hospital. Restrictions in services often have considerable consequences for older people and their carers (Littlechild and Glasby, 2000).

❖ Health Authority and other organisational purchasers, rather than service users and carers make most decisions about which services are purchased by the NHS (Pilgrim and Waldron, 1998; Ryan, 1998).

❖ Powerful banking, pharmaceutical and other interests influence the treatment alternatives available (Hogg, 1999; Stein, 1997).

❖ '... The ability of individuals to act as market consumers may be undermined by the inequality of knowledge and information... between producer and consumer...' (Lupton, 1998, p. 50).

❖ People who use health services in a crisis find it very difficult to exercise choice. This has been found, for example, in research on older people's decisions to move into residential care at the time of a crisis (Allen *et al*, 1992).

In contrast to the term 'consumers', Manos (2000) coined the term 'prosumers' to describe:

... former mental patients, graduates of various forms of living hell, transformed and activated towards a variety of work roles, focused on others who are still in the early stages of defining themselves and their beings...

(Manos, 2000, p.77)

Do service users and carers want to participate and be empowered?

For national and local health service policies on participation and empowerment to be successful, it is suggested that there needs to be recognition of the vast diversity amongst 'service users' and 'carers'; and of their views and beliefs about the delivery of care and services, and the extent that they wish to be empowered or to participate (Hogg, 1999). In some cases, there are disagreements between different groups of service users, or between the latter and carers about issues concerning service provision or policy. For example, Byrt (1994) found that the views of people with contact with mental health services ranged from total rejection to considerable acceptance and endorsement of conventional professional treatments.

The evidence suggests that service users' and carers' desired degrees and levels of participation and empowerment vary, and are influenced by many factors. These include personality factors, eg. related to locus of control (Tones and Green, 2002), previous experiences and expectations of services and of the roles of themselves and professionals (Robinson and Thomson, 2001); and their confidence and willingness to be actively involved (Byrt, 1994). Some research has found that younger people and individuals with more educational qualifications are more likely to wish to participate in medical decision making. One study found that women were more likely to wish to choose treatment. Cultural factors have also been found to be important, as is the nature and severity of the individual's illness (Florin and Coulter, 2001, Robinson and Thomson, 2001, citing various studies). The attitudes of managers and professionals, and their commitment to enabling participation and empowerment are also important (Byrt, 1994). (These and other factors facilitating and hindering empowerment and participation are considered in *Chapter 21*.)

Some critics have criticised some professionals' tendencies to assume both that it is a 'good thing' for service users to participate or to be empowered, and that they want opportunities to do so (Caress *et al*, 1998; Kendall, 1998). It is a paradox that empowerment and participation can be imposed against service users' wishes. One of the present authors is reminded of the comment of a resident in a therapeutic community where he was a charge nurse: 'I know you want us to give our views. But why should I? I don't have any say in my family or the place where I work'.

Some individuals participate in the role of 'carer', often with long hours and considerable responsibility, because of the absence of professional help, or a lack of information about appropriate services (Dearden and Becker, 2000); and not necessarily for any wish to be involved to this extent (Henwood, 1998). Even with recent central government initiatives to support carers, the amount of support they can expect is often unclear (Banks, 2001). In one study, some people with service user experience participated in voluntary organisations because of the absence of other volunteers, and not because they wished to participate (Byrt and Dooher, 2002, citing Byrt, 1994).

In relation to individual care and treatment, research indicates that the desired amount of participation and empowerment depends, in part, on the service user's preferences and the extent of his/her illness (Robinson and Thomson, 2001) or level of distress. For example, people with diagnoses of 'antisocial' and 'borderline personality disorders' often find it very difficult to trust professionals because of past adverse experience of neglect and abuse from parents and others. In addition, they are labelled with stigmatising diagnoses and often experience negative attitudes from professionals (Ashman, 2001; Castillo *et al*, 2001; Hadden and Haigh, 2001 and 2002). For these reasons, individuals with these experiences find it difficult to engage with staff or participate in treatment. It has been argued that professionals need to recognise that such clients go through various stages of treatment acceptance, including their readiness to actively participate in decisions about their care, or (in the case of therapeutic communities, see *Chapter 10*) that of others (Campling, 1999; Norton and Hinshelwood, 1996). The 'participation' of people with 'personality disorders' in secure hospitals and units is, in any case, limited because they sometimes have little choice but to receive treatment (George, 1998).

Several studies have examined the extent to which service users desire empowerment or participation. In general, research suggests that many, although not all patients would like improved communication, including more information (Evans and Byrt, 2002; Florin and Coulter, 2001, citing several studies). (Information is often seen as the lowest degree of participation: Byrt and Dooher, 2002.) Good communication is associated with service user satisfaction (Florin and Coulter, 2001). The latter authors conclude:

> *... Less is known... about the extent to which patients want to share decisions rather than just information... The age differences in decision-making preferences suggest that the preference for active involvement may be increasing over time, reflecting greater knowledge of the risks, as well as the benefits, of medical care, and decreased willingness to submit to the authority of clinicians...*

(Florin and Coulter, p. 53)

Research suggests that although many service users and carers desire more information, many do not want to participate at higher degrees, for example, in making decisions. Byrt (1994) found that many voluntary organisation members with experience of mental health problems were keen to be involved in putting forward their views and taking on responsibilities. However, few of these individuals wished to participate in running their organisation, locally or nationally. Florin and Coulter (2001) suggest that a distinction between paternalistic and 'patient-centred' models of consultations in general practice is a 'false dichotomy', since it might be appropriate to use both models with the same patient at different times, depending on his/her needs. These authors point out that some patients prefer doctors to make decisions; and that expectations that they are active participants may engender discomfort. Research has found that fewer patients with carcinomas wished to choose treatments, compared with healthy individuals who were asked if they would like such a choice if they developed cancer (Florin and Coulter, 2001, citing Degner and Sloan, 1992).

The desired amount of participation is often related to the seriousness of the health problem (Robinson and Thomson, 2001). Biley '... found that patients, if well enough, wanted full involvement in decisions in … activities of daily living...' (Biley, 1992) but did not wish to participate in areas such as 'dressings and drugs', in which they considered that the nurse knew best. According to Robinson and Thomson (2001):

> *… Degner and Sloan reported that patients close to a life threatening event were more passive with respect to treatment decisions than a comparison group of healthy individuals. In another study, … preference for handing over control to the physician was found to be significantly greater for the vignette involving potential mortality (chest pain) than for the vignettes involving mainly morbidity (urinary problems) or quality of life (fertility)...*

> (Robinson and Thomson, 2001, p. 35f,
> citing Degner and Sloan, 1992,
> and Deber *et al*, 1996)

Brashers *et al* (1999) also found that patients varied in the extent to which they wished to participate actively in their care. One group of 'AIDS patient activists' were found to be particularly active participants, as measured by a patient self-advocacy scale developed by Brashers and Klingle (1992, cited in Brashers *et al*, 1999). These individuals were found to be more assertive in their interactions with medical staff, actively searched for information and were more likely to make informed choices not to continue with prescribed treatments.

Smith and Draper measured the extent to which general hospital patients wished to have control in their care. No differences were found '... between nurse and patient perceptions of [actual] patient control...' (Smith and Draper, 1994, p. 854). However, nurses frequently made assumptions, based on their own views, that patients wanted more control than was desired by the patients themselves. Smith and Draper proposed:

> *... The development of a tool to assess the amount of control desired by patients. This would help to ensure that nursing care is congruent with the beliefs of the patient, rather than the nurse...*

(Smith and Draper, 1994, p. 854)

Degner produced a scale to measure the desired amount of participation in decisions in medical consultations, ranging from those made solely by the patient to decisions left entirely to the doctor's discretion (Degner and Sloan, 1992, cited in Robinson and Thomson, 2001, see *Box 1.1, p. 16*). While Degner's Scale can be used to assess service users' and carers' participation preferences in decision making, it does not measure their wish for information. Furthermore, individuals may not be aware of the consequences of such participation, in relation to treatment outcomes; and may have a lack of information to inform their decisions (Robinson and Thomson, 2001).

Caress *et al* (1998) compared renal patients' **preferred** roles with their perceptions of their **actual** roles in decision making about their care. Preferred and actual roles corresponded in only approximately one third of patients. Over half the respondents in this study had less involvement, and one in ten had more involvement, than they would have preferred. Caress *et al* propose that the card sort used in their research could:

> *... provide practitioners with information which could be used to facilitate the bringing of preferred and perceived roles more closely into line. For some health professionals, this might mean allowing patients a more active role in treatment decision making. For others, it might require recognition that not all patients are desirous of active participation...*

(Caress *et al*, 1998, p. 371)

Parents' wish to participate

Research on parental participation of children in hospital also suggests that the amount and type of participation desired by parents is often unrelated to what is provided or expected by staff. This includes information given to parents and professionals' expectations that they should, or should not, be involved in various aspects of their child's care (Blower and Morgan, 2000; Savage and Callery, 2000; Simons *et al*, 2001).

> *... [P]arents who lived-in with their hospitalised child... reported feeling uncertain about what was expected of them... The parents felt under pressure to participate and establish themselves in the eyes of the professionals as 'good' parents...*

(Teasdale, 1998, p. 99, citing Darbyshire, 1992)

Sawley (2002) found that parents were not keen on 'family centred care', with its emphasis on parental participation, despite the promotion of the latter in children's services. Differences between parents and nurses have also been reported in relation to their understanding of what 'parental participation' means; and their attitudes towards what Darbyshire (1996) refers to as, '... one of paediatric nursing's most amorphous and ill-described concepts...' (Darbyshire, 1996, p. 181). The literature indicates that conceptually, parental participation '... is quite complex and may be interpreted in many ways...' (Simons *et al*, 2001, p. 593).

In a review of relevant literature, Savage and Callery (2000) reported that in eleven out of sixteen studies, some parents expressed a wish for greater participation in the care of their children in hospital. However, research has also found that many parents are distressed or uncertain about their participation in practical procedures and technical aspects of care. In addition, parents may vary in their aptitudes for participation in decision making (Hallstrom *et al*, 2002). Parents' needs to receive more information and greater professional recognition of their expert knowledge and experience of their child and his/her needs have also been highlighted (Blower and Morgan, 2000; Savage and Callery, 2000; Simons *et al*, 2000). Studies have found that, compared with nurses, parents can assess their hospitalised children's pain more accurately, but despite this, they are often given few opportunities for participation in this area (Simons *et al*, 2001, citing several studies).

Research by Simons *et al* revealed parents' frustration at the lack of an active role in managing their children's pain. Although most nurses and parents considered that there was some parental participation in this area, this was generally limited, with parents playing passive roles, and, in some cases, receiving inadequate information. Parents were not invited to participate, and there was an absence of partnership or nurse-initiated 'discussion or negotiation of the role of parents' (Simons *et al*, 2001, p. 594). The lack of negotiation with parents has been found in several other studies (Savage and Callery, 2000). The authors suggest that the possibility of participation should be discussed with parents when children are admitted, with the development of strategies to facilitate such involvement. A number of researchers have used qualitative methods or devised tools, including Likert rating scales, to assess patient participation (Savage and Callery, 2000, citing Jones, 1994; Schepp, 1992; Tomlinson *et al*, 1993 and other authors). The following comments have relevance to the participation of other carers and service users:

> *... While... studies support a planned and shared approach to implementing parental participation... parents differ in their need to participate... What may be desirable and acceptable to one parent may be undesirable and unacceptable for another. This suggests that nurses would be well advised to pay particular attention to the individual needs of parents in order to avoid the negative consequences of... participation... In this way, parents could choose their level of participation... relative to their emotional needs, their role expectations and other commitments, their need for control and decision making, and their levels of knowledge and competence...*

(Savage and Callery, 2000, p. 71)

Stages of participation and empowerment

Finally, service users' and carers' wish to participate and be empowered may vary, according to the extent of their experience of a particular illness or disability. A number of authors have outlined different **stages** of participation, both in individual care and in decisions about services and policies (Brach *et al*, 1999; Kelson,

1997; Sanoff, 2000; Smithies and Webster, 1998). Many service users and carers prefer gradually to increase their level and degree of participation. Sometimes this develops with increasing confidence and experience, as found by Gibson (1995) in her study of mothers of children with long term neurological problems, and outlined in Byrt and Dooher (2002) and Teasdale (1998). In contrast, most studies of 'knowledge' of diabetes, in individuals with this condition, have found that this decreases with increasing age and experience of the diabetes (Gillibrand and Flynn, 2001). The possible reasons for this (including professionals' discounting service users' own knowledge and experience) are considered in Byrt and Dooher, 2002.

Users of a service, who, sadly, have previously been offered little choice, may find opportunities to participate, or to be empowered, bewildering. They may feel more comfortable if participation and empowerment are introduced at the individual level with opportunities to make choice and decisions about their lives (Sayce, 2000). In addition, it may be easier for such people, at least at first, to participate through information and consultation processes, rather than through direct involvement in decision making and responsibility in the running of an organisation or in wider policy making. (However, some critics have criticised information and consultation as constituting 'pseudo-participation' or 'tokenism': Byrt and Dooher, 2002). It is suggested, in line with the research cited above, that managers and professionals need to ask service users the extent to which they wish to participate, rather than make assumptions about this. In one mental health day centre run by a voluntary organisation, various levels and degrees of participation were available, but members were not pressured to participate if they did not wish to do so (Byrt, 1994).

Accounts of stages of participation include outlines of ways in which health service users' involvement can be facilitated at all stages of research projects on patients' views (Kelson, 1997; Kemshall and Littlechild, 2000). This includes determining the scope and questions used in surveys, decisions about research method, participating in interviewing other service users, making recommendations and, '... monitoring how the recommendations are translated into practice...' (Kelson, 1997, p. 17). Smithies and Webster (1998) describe community participation in needs assessments of local communities and Sanoff (2000) outlines stages of participation in urban planning and related areas.

Bracht *et al* (1999) delineate five stages of community organisation in developing health promotion: community analysis, design initiation, implementation, maintenance — consolidation and dissemination — and re-assessment. These authors, citing Nix (1978), refer to the need to recognise both resistance and readiness to change, in addition to the identification of various factors or skills to facilitate partnership and coalitions with people involved in various agencies (Bracht *et al*, 1999). Stages of participation and gradually increased involvement in community projects are discussed in *Chapter 19* and in Tones and Green 2002 (in Dooher and Byrt, 2002).

Conclusion

The extent that 'service users' and 'carers' are empowered or able to participate depends, in part, on the relative amounts of power of the many other stakeholders in health services, and their willingness to share this. A wide range of terms has been used to describe 'service users'. These partly reflect the extent that individuals have chosen, or been compelled, to use services; the extent of their empowerment and participation; and their relationships with professionals. Some terms reflect the priorities of governments, managers or professionals, rather than those of 'service users' and 'carers'. As an example, the word 'consumer' reflects market ideologies that do not accord with the views of some clients/patients and the (usually limited) choices available to them. Many individuals described as 'carers' do not perceive themselves in this way. It is important to appreciate the diversity of 'service users' and 'carers', including variation, indicated by research findings, in the extent that they wish to participate and be empowered; and in their desired type, level and degree of participation. Ways of assessing this have been proposed, to ensure congruence between individuals' desire to participate and the opportunities provided, with some individuals preferring these to be gradually increased. Studies indicate that many individuals would like improved information and other aspects of communication from professionals. Finally, some authors have identified stages of empowerment and participation in care, services and research projects.

Some of the above themes are considered in the next chapter in relation to individuals who choose, or are compelled to use, mental health services.

Key points

❊ The extent of empowerment and participation of 'service users' and 'carers' is influenced by the relative amounts of power of many other stakeholders in health services. These include various powerful individuals and organisations, including the Department of Health, politicians, professionals and managers; and, in particular, commercial interests.

❊ Various terms have been used to describe users of health services. Such terms reflect the status of these individuals. A wide range of individuals can be considered 'service users'.

❊ Terms to describe service users include those imposed by professionals, or by wider society; and, in some instances, challenged by service users as being stigmatising. Other terms such as 'survivor', are chosen by service users themselves.

❊ The term 'carer' has been criticised for not reflecting the complexity and reciprocity of relationships involved. However, the use of this word has enable individuals so described to raise their public and political visibility. Recent legislation has considered carers and their needs.

❊ The diversity of carers and their varied needs, other roles and expertise have not always been recognised. Professionals have often failed to provide adequate information and opportunities for consultation and partnership.

❊ Researchers have proposed models of professional-service user relationships. These range from professionals' control of decision making to service users having total control and autonomy.

❊ Recently, many health service participants have argued for care and treatment approaches and professional-service user/carer relationships that involve partnership or active participation.

❊ People who pay for services are consumers in the economic sense. From 1979, under Conservative and to some extent, New Labour governments, there has been an increasing emphasis on the health service user as 'consumer'.

❊ However, critics have argued that consumerist participation, especially choice, is limited in health services, particularly for people unable to afford private treatment and care, or who need to make choices at a time of crisis.

✻ Research suggests that service users and carers vary in their views of services and the extent that they wish to participate. This is related to several factors. There is evidence that many service users and carers would like more information and improved communication from professionals.

✻ Service users'/carers' desired levels and degrees of participation, and ways to participate need to be assessed, with opportunities to participate being tailored to the wishes of the individual. Several tools have been devised to assess desired participation.

✻ Participation and empowerment can occur at different stages of policy making, care and service provision and research. Individual and community participation and empowerment may take time to develop, and some service users may prefer these to be gradually increased.

References

Allen I, Hogg D, Peace S (1992) *Elderly People. Choice, Participation and Satisfaction.* Policy Studies Institute, London

Andershed B, Ternestedt B-M (2001) Development of a theoretical framework describing relatives' involvement in palliative care. *J Adv Nurs* **34**(4): 554–62

Anderson W (2001) Primary care groups: corporate opportunities for public involvement. In: Gillam S, Brooks F, eds. *New Beginnings. Towards Patient and Public Involvement.* King's Fund/University of Luton, London

Ashman D (2001) Desperately seeking understanding. *Mental Health Today* October: 30–1

Banks P (2001) Carers' contribution in primary care. In: Gillam S, Brooks F, eds. *New Beginnings. Towards Patient and Public Involvement in Primary Health Care.* King's Fund/University of Luton, London

Barker P (1999) *The Philosophy and Practice of Psychiatric Nursing.* Churchill Livingstone, Edinburgh

Barnes M (1997) Families and empowerment. In: Ramcharan P, Roberts G, Grant G, Borland J, eds. *Empowerment in Everyday Life. Learning Disability.* Jessica Kingsley, London

Barnes M, Warren L, eds (1999) *Paths to Empowerment.* The Policy Press, University of Bristol, Bristol

Barnes M, Bowl R (2001) *Taking Over the Asylum.* Palgrave, Basingstoke

Biley FC (1992) Some determinants that affect patient participation in decision making about nursing care. *J Adv Nurs* **15**(1): 27–37

Blower K, Morgan E (2000) Great Expectations? Parental participation in care. *J Child Health Care* **4**(2): 60–5

Bracht N, Kingsbury L, Rissel C (1999) A Five-Stage Community Organisation Model for Health Promotion. In: Bracht N, ed. *Health Promotion at the Community Level. 2. New Advances.* Sage Publications, Thousand Oaks: chapter 4

Brager G, Specht H, TorczynerJL (1987) *Community Organising.* 2nd edn. Columbia University Press, New York

Brandon D (1981) *Voices of Experience.* MIND Publications, London

Brashers DE *et al* (1999) The patient self-advocacy scale: measuring patient involvement in health care decision — making interactions. *Health Communications* **11**(2): 97–121

Braye S (2000) Participation and involvement in social care: an overview. In: Kemshall H, Littlechild R *op cit*: chapter 2

Brooks F (2001) Why user involvement in primary health care? In: Gillam S, Brooks F, eds. *New Beginnings. Towards Patient and Public Involvement in Primary Health Care*. King's Fund/University of Luton, London

Brooks F, Gillam S (2001) Preface. In: Gillam S, Brooks F, eds. *New Beginnings. Towards Patient and Public Involvement in Primary Health Care*. King's Fund/University of Luton, London

Bucknall O, Holmes G (2001) Relatives and carers. In: Newnes C, Holmes G, Dunn C *op cit*: chapter 12

Butler D (1998) Foreword. In: Warner L, Wexler S (1998) *Eight Hours a Day and Taken for Granted?* Research Commissioned by The Princess Royal Trust for Carers. The Princess Royal Trust for Carers, London

Butler L (2002) Empowerment and participation: the arts in healthcare.In: Dooher J, Byrt , eds. *Empowerment and participation: power, influence and control in contemporary health care*. Quay Books, Mark Allen Publishing Limited, Salisbury: chapter 14

Byrt R (1994) *Consumer Participation in a Voluntary Organisation for Mental Health*. Unpublished PhD Thesis, Loughborough University, Loughborough

Byrt R (2000) Dangerous proposals? A response to 'managing dangerous people with personality disorder'. *Mental Health Practice* 3(10): 12–17

Byrt R (2001) Power, influence and control in practice development. In: Clark A, Dooher J, Fowler J, eds. *The Handbook of Practice Development*. Quay Books, Mark Allen Publishing Limited, Salisbury: chapter 10

Byrt R, Dooher J (2002) Empowerment and participation: definitions, meanings and models. In: Dooher J, Byrt R, eds. *op cit*: chapter 2

Cameron A (1999) The role of interest groups. In: Masterson A, Maslin-Prothero S, eds. *Nursing and Politics. Power Through Practice*. Churchill Livingstone, Edinburgh: chapter 4

Campbell P (1998) Listening to Clients. In: Barker P, Davidson B, eds. *Psychiatric Nursing. Ethical Strife*. Arnold, London: chapter 17

Campling P (1999) Chaotic personalities. Maintaining the therapeutic alliance. In: Campling P, Haigh R, eds. *Therapeutic Communities. Past, Present and Future*. Jessica Kingsley, London: chapter 11

Caress AL *et al* (1998) Patient-sensitive treatment decision making? Preferences and perceptions of a sample of renal patients. *NT Research* 3(5): 364–72

Castillo H, Allen L, Coxhead N (2001) The hurtfulness of a diagnosis: user research on personality disorder. *Mental Health Practice* 4(9): 16–19

Chamberlin J (1988) *On Our Own. Patient Controlled Alternatives to the Mental Health System*. MIND Publications, London

Chamberlin J (2000) The medical model and harm. In: Barker P, Campbell P, Davidson B, eds. *From the Ashes of Experience. Reflections on Madness, Survival and Growth*. Whurr Publishers, London: chapter 11

Chiu S, Yu S (2001) An excess of culture: the myth of shared care in the Chinese community in Britain. *Ageing and Society* **21**: 681–99

Clayton J (1998) Caring in a Mixed Economy. In: Birchenall M, Birchenall P, eds. *Sociology as Applied to Nursing and Health Care*. Baillière Tindall in association with the Royal College of Nursing, London: chapter 11

Corker M, Davis JM (2000) Disabled children: (still) invisible under the law. In: Cooper J, ed. *Law, Rights and Disability*. Jessica Kingsley, London: chapter 10

Darbyshire P (1996) Parents, nurses and paediatric nursing: A Critical Review. In: Smith JP, ed. *Nursing Care of Children*. Blackwell Science, Oxford: chapter 12

Dearden C, Becker S (2000) Listening to children: meeting the needs of young carers. In: Kemshall H, Littlechild R *op cit*

Deborah (1999) *Informing Relatives and Partners about Personality Disorder?* Dialogue. Newsletter of the Virtual Institute of Severe Personality Disorder. No 3, Winter 1999/2000: 5

Department of Health (1991) *The Patient's Charter*. DoH, London

Department of Health (1996a) Carers (Recognition and Services) Act 1995. HMSO, London

Department of Health (1996b) *The Patient's Charter and You*. DoH, London

Department of Health (1997a) *The new NHS — modern, dependable*. DoH, London

Department of Health (1997b) *The Patient's Charter. Mental Health Services*. DoH, London

Department of Health (1998) *A First Class Service: Quality in the New NHS*. DoH, London

Department of Health (1999) *National Service Framework for Mental Health*. DoH, London

Department of Health (2000a) *The NHS Cancer Plan: a plan for investment, a plan for reform*. DoH, London

Department of Health (2000b) *The NHS Plan. A Plan for Investment. A Plan for Reform*. DoH, London

Department of Health (2001a) *Family Matters. Counting Families In*. DoH, London

Department of Health (2001b) *National Service Framework for Older People*. DoH, London

Department of Health (2002) *Communicating with Patients, Carers and Relatives, Staff and Teams. Outputs of Workshop, 22 January, 2002*. Prepared for the Department of Health by Stanton Marris. Department of Health, Leeds

Department of Health and Social Security (1983) *The NHS Management Report*. (The Griffiths Report). DHSS, London

Dooher J, Byrt, R, eds (2002) *Empowerment and Participation: Power, influence and control in contemporary health care*. Quay Books, Mark Allen Publishing Limited, Salisbury

Ellis-Hill C, Payne S (2001) The future: interventions and conceptual issues. In: Payne S, Ellis-Hill C, eds. *Chronic and Terminal Illness. New Perspectives on Caring and Carers*. Oxford University Press, Oxford: chapter 9

Evans S, Byrt R (2002) The power to complain? In: Dooher J, Byrt R *op cit*: chapter 15

Florin D, Coulter A (2001) Partnership in the primary care consultation. In: Gillam S, Brooks F, eds. *New Beginnings. Towards Patient and Public Involvement in Primary Health Care*. King's Fund/University of Luton, London: chapter 4

George S (1998) 'More than a pound of flesh: A patient's perspective'. In: Mason T, Mercer S, *op cit*: chapter 7

Gibson CH (1995) The process of empowerment in mothers of chronically disabled children. *J Adv Nurs* **21**: 1201–10

Gillibrand W, Flynn M (2001) Forced externalization of control in people with diabetes: a qualitative exploratory study. *J Adv Nurs* **34**(4): 501–10

Godsell M (1999) Caring for people with learning disabilities. In: Wilkinson G, Miers M, eds. *Power and Nursing Practice*. Macmillan, Basingstoke: chapter 14

Godfrey J (1999) Empowerment through sexuality. In: Wilkinson G, Miers M, eds. *Power and Nursing Practice*. Macmillan, Basingstoke: chapter 12

Hadden Y, Haigh R (2001) *Personality disorder — how much more stigmatising could a label be? Part 1. Dialogue*. Virtual Institute of Severe Personality Disorder Newsletter. No 9, Winter: 1–2

Hadden Y, Haigh R (2002) *Personality Disorder — how much more stigmatising could a label be? Part 2. Dialogue*. Virtual Institute of Severe Personality Disorder Newsletter. No 10, Spring: 1–2

Hallstom I, Runeson I, Elander G (2002) An observational study of the level at which parents participate in decisions during their child's hospitalization. *Nurs Ethics* **9**(2): 202–14

Ham C (1985) *State of the Art*. In: Centre Eight. Consumerism in the NHS. *Health and Social Service J* **94**(4950) Supplement: 1–2

Handy CB (1993) *Understanding Organizations*. 2nd edn. Penguin Books, Harmondsworth

Heaphy B, Weeks J, Donovan C (1999) Narratives of care, love and commitment: AIDS/HIV and non-heterosexual family formations. In: Aggleton P, Hart G, Davies P, eds. *Families and Communities Responding to AIDS*. UCL Press/Taylor and Francis Group, London: chapter 5

Henwood M (1998) *Ignored and Invisible? Carers' Experience of the NHS. Report of a UK Research Survey Commissioned by Carers National Association*. Carers National Association, London

HM Government (1997) *The new NHS — modern, dependable*. Command 3807. DoH, London

Heron C (1998) *Working with Carers*. Jessica Kingsley, London

Hogg C (1999) *Patients, Power and Politics. From Patients to Citizens*. Sage, London

Hunt P, Reynolds MA (1985) Challenges to Health Authorities. In: Centre 8: *Consumerism in the NHS. Health and Social Service J* **94**(4950), Supplement: 7–8

Jones C (1994) Effect of parental participation on hospitalised child behavior. *Issues in Comprehensive Pediatric Nursing* **17**: 81–92. Cited in: Savage E, Callery P (2000) *op cit*

Jones K (1993) *Asylums and after. A revised history of the mental health services: from the early eighteenth century to the nineteen nineties*. The Athlone Press, London

Kelson M (1997) *User involvement. A guide to developing effective user involvement strategies in the NHS*. College of Health, London

Kemshall H, Littlechild R, eds (2000) *User Involvement and Participation in Social Care. Research Informing Practice*. Jessica Kingsley, London

Kendall S (1998) Introduction. In: Kendall S, ed. *Health and Empowerment. Research and Practice*. Arnold, London

Kennard D (1998) *An Introduction to Therapeutic Communities*. Jessica Kingsley, London

Klein R (1973) *Complaints Against Doctors.* Charles Knight, London

Kohner N, Hill A, eds (2000) *Help! Does My Patient Know More than Me?* King's Fund, London

Lilley P (2000) *Patient Power. Choice for a Better NHS.* Demos, London

Littlechild R, Glasby J (2000) Older people as 'participating patients'. In: Kemshall H, Littlechild R, eds. *op cit:* chapter 9

Lupton C (1998) *Managing Public Involvement in Healthcare Purchasing.* Open University Press, Aylesbury

McFadyen J, Farrington A (1997) User and carer participation in the NHS. *Br J Health Care Management* **3**(5): 260–4

Manos E (2000) The Flight of the Phoenix. In: Barker P, Campbell P, Davidson B, eds. *From the Ashes of Experience. Reflections on Madness, Survival and Growth.* Whurr Publishers, London: chapter 5

Martin J, Evans D (1984) *Hospitals in Trouble.* Blackwell, Oxford

Mason T, Mercer D, eds (1998) *Critical Perspectives in Forensic Care. Inside Out.* Macmillan, Basingstoke

May J, Ellis-Hill C, Payne S (2001) Gatekeeping and legitimization: How informal carers' relationship with health care workers is revealed in their everyday interactions. *J Adv Nurs* **36**(3): 364–75

Miers M (1999) Involving clients in decision making: Breast care nursing. In: Wilkinson G, Miers M, eds. *Power and Nursing Practice.* Macmillan, Basingstoke: chapter 13

Mind Out for Mental Health (Undated) *Postcard.* MIND, London

Newnes C, Holmes G, Dunn C, eds (2001) *This is Madness Too. Critical Perspectives on Mental Health Services.* PCCS Books, Ross on Wye

Nolan M, Grant G, Keady J (1995) Developing a typology of family care: implications for nurses and other service providers. *J Adv Nurs* **21**: 256–65. Cited in: Payne S, Ellis-Hill C (2001) *op cit*

Nolan M (2001) Positive aspects of caring. In: Payne S, Ellis-Hill C, eds. *Chronic and Terminal Illness. New Perspectives on Caring and Carers.* Oxford University Press, Oxford: chapter 2

Norton K, Hinshelwood RD (1996) Severe personality disorder: treatment issues and selection for inpatient psychotherapy. *Br J Psychiatry* **168**(6): 723–31

Oliver M, Barnes C (1998) *Disabled People and Social Policy.* Longman, London

Patel N, Fatimilehin IA (1999) Racism and mental health. In: Newnes C, Holmes G, Dunn C, eds. *This is Madness. A Critical Look at Psychiatry and the Future of Mental Health Services.* PCCS Books, Ross on Wye: chapter 3

Paterson B (2001) Myth of empowerment in chronic illness. *J Adv Nurs* **34**(5): 574–81

Payne S, Ellis-Hill C (2001) Being a carer. In: Payne S, Ellis-Hill C, eds. *Chronic and Terminal Illness. New Perspectives on Caring and Carers.* Oxford University Press, Oxford: chapter 1

Pilgrim D, Waldron L (1998) User involvement in mental health service developments. How far can it go? *J Mental Health* **1**(1): 95–104

Porter R, ed (1991) *The Faber Book of Madness.* Faber and Faber, London

Preston-Shoot M (2000) Clear Voices for Change: Messages from Disability Research for Law, Policy and Practice. In: Cooper J, ed. *Law, Rights and Disability.* Jessica Kingsley, London: chapter 11

Priestley M (1999) *Disability Politics and Community Care.* Jessica Kingsley, London

Prior PM (1999) *Gender and Mental Health.* Macmillan, Basingstoke

Robinson A, Thompson R (2001) Variability in patient preferences for participating in medical decision making: implication for the use of decision support tools. *Quality in Health Care* **10**(supplement I): i34–i38

Rogers H (2000) Breaking the ice. Developing strategies for collaborative working with carers of older people with mental health problems. In: Kemshall H, Littlechild, eds. *op cit:* chapter 7

Royal College of Physicians of London and College of Health (1998) *Stroke Rehabilitation Patient and Carer Views. A Report from the Intercollegiate Working Party for Stroke.* Royal College of Physicians, London: November

Royal Commission on the NHS (1979) *A Service for Patients. Conclusions and Recommendation of the Royal Commission's Report (Merrison Report).* HMSO, London: July

Ryan S (1998) Disadvantaged Groups in Health Care. In: Birchenall M, Birchenall P, eds. *Sociology as applied to nursing and health care.* Baillière and Tindall in association with the Royal College of Nursing, London: chapter 6

Saks M (2002) Empowerment, participation and the rise of orthodox biomedicine. In: Dooher J, Byrt R, eds. *op cit:* chapter 3

Salman S (2002) Bullying Tactics. *The Guardian,* Society Supplement: 3 April, 56–5

Sanoff H (2000) *Community Participation. Methods in Design and Planning.* John Wiley, New York

Savage E, Callery P (2000) Parental participation in the care of hospitalised children. A review of the evidence. In: Glasper AE, Ireland L, eds. *Evidence-Based Child Health Care. Challenges for Practice.* Macmillan Press Limited, Basingstoke: chapter 5

Sawley L (2002) Consumer groups: sharing education and developing practice. *Paediatric Nurs* **14**(3): 18–21

Sayce L (2000) *From Psychiatric Patient to Citizen. Overcoming Discrimination and Social Exclusion.* Macmillan, Basingstoke

Schepp K (1992) Correlates of mothers who prefer control over their hospitalised children's care. *J Paediatr Nurs* **7**(2): 83–9. Cited in: Savage E, Callery P (2000) *op cit*

Simons J, Franck L, Roberson E (2001) Parent involvement in children's pain care: views of parents and nurses. *J Adv Nurs* **36**(4): 591–9

Smith J (1987) Social Services. In: Clode D, Parker C, Etherington S, eds. *Towards the Sensitive Bureaucracy, Consumers, Welfare and the New Pluralism.* Gower, Aldershot

Smith R, Draper P (1994) 'Who is in Control? An Investigation of Nurse and Patient Beliefs Relating to Control of their Health Care'. *J Adv Nurs* **19**: 884–92

Smithies J, Webster G (1998) *Community Involvement in Health. From Passive Recipients to Active Participants.* Ashgate, Aldershot

Spurgeon P, Smith P, Straker M, Deakin N, Thomas N, Walsh K (1997) The experience of contracting in health care. In: Flynn R, Williams G, eds. *Contracting for Health. Quasi-Markets and the National Health Service.* Oxford University Press, Oxford: chapter 9

Stein J (1997) *Empowerment and Women's Health. Theory, Methods and Practice.* Zed Books, London

Sturt J (1998) Implementing theory into primary health care practice; an empowering approach. In: Kendall S, ed. *Health and Empowerment Research and Practice.* Arnold, London

Survivors' Poetry Scotland (1996) *Sweet, Sour and Serious. Illustrated Anthology.* Survivors' Press Glasgow

Tannsjo T (1999) *Coercive Care. The Ethics of Choice in Health and Medicine.* Routledge, London

Taylor S (1999) *Health Psychology.* 4th edn. McGraw-Hill, Boston

Teasdale K (1998) *Advocacy in Health Care.* Blackwell Science, Oxford

Tomlinson P, Kirschawm M, Tomczyk B, Peterson J (1993) The relationship of child acuity: maternal responses, nurses' attitudes and contextual factors in the bone marrow transplant unit. *Am J Crit Care* **2**(3): 246–7

Tones K (1998) Empowerment for health: the challenge. In: Kendall S, ed. *Health and Empowerment. Research and Practice.* Arnold, London: chapter 9

Tones K, Green J (2002) The empowerment imperative in health promotion. In: Dooher J, Byrt R, eds. *op cit*: chapter 5

Twig J, Atkin K (1994) *Carers Perceived.* Open University Press, Buckingham

United Kingdom Central Council for Nursing, Midwifery and Health Visiting (1999) *Nursing in Secure Environments. A Summary.* UKCC, London

Wakefield T (1983) *Mates.* GMP, London

Walker E, Dewar BJ (2001) How do we facilitate carers' involvement in decision making? *J Adv Nurs* **34**(3): 329–37

Wallcraft J, Michaelson J (2001) Developing a survivor discourse to replace the 'psychopathology' of breakdown and crisis. In: Newnes C, Holmes G, Dunn C, eds. *op cit*: chapter 16

Walmsley J, Downer J (1997) Shouting the loudest: self-advocacy, power and diversity. In: Ramcharan P, Roberts G, Grant G, Borland J, eds. *Empowerment in Everyday Life. Learning Disability.* Jessica Kingsley, London: chapter 3

Warren L (1999) Conclusion. Empowerment: the path to partnership? In: Barnes M, Warren L, eds. *Paths to Empowerment.* The Policy Press, University of Bristol, Bristol: 119–143

Webb R, Tossell D (1999) *Social Issues for Carers. Towards Positive Practice.* 2nd edn. Arnold, London

Wilton T (2000) *Sexualities in Health and Social Care: A textbook.* Open University Press, Buckingham

Windle C, Cibulka JG (1981) A framework for understanding participation in community mental health services. *Community Mental Health J* **17**: Part 1

Wright A (1999) Exploring the Development of User Forums in an NHS Trust. In: Barnes M, Warren L, eds. *Paths to Empowerment.* The Policy Press, University of Bristol, Bristol: 51–67

2

User empowerment and user involvement in mental health

Ann Jackson and John Hyslop

Introduction

This chapter will examine the establishment of 'user-involvement' as viable, both conceptually and in its practical implementation within the arena of mental health. We will seek to consider the inherent difficulties associated with an approach that can be interpreted as anything from tokenistic 'consultation' to the explicit demands of some factions of the user movement for 'empowerment'.

The term 'empowerment' is itself without clarity and is reflective of a wider and problematic discourse. This discussion draws on sociological perspectives as applied generally to health, and more specifically to 'empowerment' as realised, or not, within mental health policy and research. What might be seen as 'empowerment' to one person, to another would be no more than a gesture of 'giving voice'. Determining the scope for ('true') empowerment involves a re-examination of those values that can be tangibly associated with individual roles and actions that operate in order to influence the state in which another might, or might not be, 'empowered' (Zarb, 1992).

Different approaches to empowerment have been influenced by the different theoretical and practical contexts in which the debates have taken place. 'User involvement' may be perceived as desirable from consumerist, medical, citizenship, academic or service users own (political) perspectives — all with different associated goals. The development of user-involvement as a theme within mental health services owes something to each of these debates.

For the purposes of this chapter, 'empowerment' is the ultimate goal against which other initiatives can be assessed. A useful starting point is to give a definition of 'empowerment'. Grace suggests the following:

> ... to mean the notion of people having power to take

action to control and enhance their own lives, and the processes of enabling them to do so.

(Grace, 1991, p. 330)

It is useful to highlight the special difficulties associated with 'user-involvement' in mental health. The origin and present organisation of mental health services has as its base the management of 'deviant' behaviours. Even within mainstream health care, there is scope for conflicts of interest between individual members of the public and the public as a whole. Clarke and Stewart (1997) highlight several dilemmas that can occur as a result of local authorities attempting to reconcile the different needs (and interests) of the 'public' as customer, citizen and community. Within mental health, there are additional special difficulties which result from a perception among the public of risk violence at the hands of psychiatric patients, and a corresponding perceived risk amongst 'psychiatric patients' of risk of violence at the hands of the psychiatric system.

A history of 'user-involvement'

It is useful to consider the historical context from which this debate emerges. Since the 1950s, sociologists have recognised that 'illness' can be described and interpreted as a social role as well as a medical condition (Parsons, 1951). The loss of 'normal' functioning, the consequent loss of independence and potential threat to individual identity are still central concepts in attempts to understand the perils of 'illness' for an individual (Nettleton, 1995). These perils are amplified if the 'illness' is considered to be mental, as the scope for forced detention, treatment and social stigma is potentially greater. This was recognised by the deviance theorists and members of the so-called 'anti-psychiatry' movement during the 1960s (see Sedgewick, 1982, for a critique of this term). From a collection of widely differing theoretical critiques, the unifying theme was the alleged oppressive nature of psychiatry, and consequent 'disempowerment' of the psychiatric patient.

The themes espoused by the 'anti-psychiatrists', initially widely dismissed, gained some credence following a series of high-profile scandals concerning the brutal treatment of psychiatric patients during the early 1970s. It is not the intention here to suggest that this is where the sympathies of all activist groups currently lie. Overt 'anti-psychiatry' principles are often still dismissed by those with vested interests and power, and as Campbell (1996) suggests, some groups are taking a 'post-psychiatric' approach that might be more politically viable. However, the historical importance of anti-psychiatry lay in the development of an arena in which user-involvement could be debated.

The political organisation of people perceived as 'mad', or 'mentally ill' can be traced back to the industrial revolution, although without producing a sustained political edifice until the 1980s (Crane, 1998). In the context of disability, Croft and Beresford (1992) describe the developmental process. Firstly, that these groups 'experience institutionalised social oppression(s)'. Secondly, that they 'recognise and value their own particular history and culture.' Thirdly, that they 'frame their activities in political terms'. Fourthly, that they positively assert their identity. And finally, that they 'take a pride in who they are' (Croft and Beresford, 1992). Early examples of political organisation in mental health, such as the Mental Patients Union and the Campaign Against Psychiatric Oppression, clearly reflect this process. In the late 1980s, Survivors Speak Out became the first effective national voice for service users.

The 1970s and 1980s, saw a growth in the political organisation of people labelled as mentally ill, and of the perception that psychiatric services could be experienced as oppressive. Many different interest groups have subsequently sought to redress some of the evident problems in the system by focusing on the balance of power between the psychiatric patient and those designated as responsible for her or his treatment and care. Since the early 1970s, people labelled as 'mentally ill' have made considerable progress in legitimising their struggle for increased control over their interactions with mental health services. But to what extent has this legitimacy been gained at the expense of the reality of 'empowerment'? And how helpful or harmful are the recent bureaucratic developments within the National Health Service in moving towards this objective? (NHS, 1999 and 2000).

Health policy initiatives and consumerism

Many moves towards 'user-involvement' have been aligned to a consumerist intention, culminating in the NHS and Community Care Act (1990). The move towards regarding the mentally ill 'patient' as a 'consumer' or 'user' of mental health services can be traced to the 'new right' political faction of the Conservative Party, and the legislation it introduced after it came to power in 1979. Their well-known ideological commitment to a 'free market' economy was complemented by the political necessity of controlling public spending, in the NHS as much as any other area of delivery. As a result of the publication of the *Report of the National Health Service Management Committee* (1983), chaired by Sir Roy Griffiths, the NHS adopted a new management structure to replace the old inter-disciplinary teams. Managers were appointed on short-term contracts to meet targets set by a politically appointed executive. Despite the rhetoric of 'taking the politics out of the NHS', the effect was to make health authorities more politically accountable to the Government (Paton, 1990).

The next phase followed an unsuccessful attempt to broach the privatisation of the NHS at the 1986 Conservative Party Conference. John Moore, then Health Secretary, suggested a system of 'discounts' on National Insurance contributions for those willing to take out private health insurance. The Labour Party appealed to public loyalty to the NHS, and Prime Minister Margaret Thatcher moved to diffuse the issue. She replaced Moore with Kenneth Clarke, and instigated what was to become known as 'The Prime Minister's Review of the NHS', which resulted in the publication of the White Paper, *Working For Patients*, in 1989. Based around the theories of Professor Alain Enthoven, the paper introduced the concept of the 'purchaser-provider split': the health service would be divided into two, one half purchasing services for patients, the other competing with one another for contracts to provide services. The stated aim was 'to extend patient choice, to delegate responsibility to where services are provided and to secure the best value for money'. It also fulfilled the function of movement towards privatisation, by allowing the public purse to be used to purchase private services.

The rhetoric of extended consumer choice quickly came under attack, from the pro-market right wing as well as the political left. While the latter suspected cost-cutting as the ultimate objective, the former condemned the fact that budgets had not actually been devolved to patients, meaning that there was in fact no greater choice for the individual (Green, 1990). Whether this choice is falsely implied or actualised within the health care arena, 'choice' on its own will arguably not impact change on the position of the individual in relation to the service, or in effecting a wider social or political change. Grace (1991) illustrates this limitation:

> *This construction precludes a transformation of health-*
> *related social processes that could result from the*
> *challenge of health movements. ... It is ironic that a*
> *discourse [of empowerment] articulating a concern to*
> *promote health in the name of freedom and 'wholeness'*
> *functions to alienate people from their capacity to engage*
> *in protest, and effectively operates to subject them further*
> *to the political and economic order.*

(Grace, 1991, p. 341)

An interesting counterpoint to this argument is an American study of 'consumer empowerment', where the political dimension of empowerment within a consumerist role is made explicit (McLean, 1995). In describing this fusion between 'empowerment' and 'consumerism', McLean (1995) goes on to suggest that a common goal of participation, notwithstanding some important, although often subtle, political differences, is two-fold. Firstly, she identifies 'the shared feeling of disenfranchisement and powerlessness'; and secondly, 'an endorsement of the principles of self-determination and control'. Thus, a 'consumer empowerment' model represents a rejection of the abuses of mental health and at the same time demands treatment choices.

The consumerist model continued to be promulgated through the Mental Health Patient's Charter and Local Voices, a policy aimed at encouraging purchasers to consult with local communities. Not only was this policy ineffective (an NHS Executive survey concluded that only 21% of consultations were 'good'), but questionable from the perspective of empowerment, as it conflated the interests of the general public with that of service users. While there is potential overlap between these perspectives, there is also much scope for conflict (Rhodes and Nocon, 1998). This can be argued as being particularly likely in the case of mental health, where public desire for 'risky' behaviour to be managed can directly militate against the freedom of 'patients'.

Paton is more generally critical of the role of consultation, stating that the result of local consultations with the public prior to the formation of NHS trusts was that they invariably didn't want them, but the outcome was nevertheless that the plans went ahead. His perception is that the primary purpose of such consultations is to bestow legitimacy, citing a survey of forty health authorities of which only two '... differed from the view that public consultation was primarily designed to legitimise actions which were intended in any case' (Paton, 1998, p. 141).

In this context, consultation clearly does not fit Grace's (1991) criteria for empowerment. Indeed, some organisational theorists have gone so far as to argue that:

> *... through participation those in charge know more readily how to get what they want with less trouble, and those without real power still do not understand all that is being done. Indeed, those in power may become more powerful.*

(Hickson and McCullough, 1980)

New Labour and citizens' rights

The 'third way' championed by the 'New' Labour Party, both in opposition and in power, was heavily influenced by European developments. Rather than focusing on redistribution of resources as the solution to the problems of disabled people, the 'third way' emphasises the importance of 'social inclusion' and 'citizenship'. On coming to power in May 1997, the Labour Party announced a ministerial task force to examine these issues in relation to disabled people. A White Paper, published in July 1998, eventually resulted in the Disability Rights Commission Bill, which was duly enacted and set up the Commission in April 2000. The main purpose of the commission is to promote equality of opportunity and eliminate discrimination, utilising both the Disability Discrimination Act 1995 and the European rights incorporated into UK law by the Human Rights Act (1998).

The actual consequences for mental health service delivery are currently far from clear. Some sections of the 'user movement' have previously cited the 'splitting' of users of different services as a barrier to effective involvement (Lindow and Morris, 1995), while other commentators have long argued that a rights-based approach is likely to yield better results than any level of 'consultation' (Forbes and Sashidharan, 1997). However, the heavy reliance on a legal framework (for example, with respect to employment tribunals) depends on an individual's ability to gain access to legal support and advice — a problematic area for many users of mental health services.

Another criticism of the 'citizenship' debate lies in the limited scope with which politicians are interpreting it. The closeness between concepts of 'social exclusion' and 'exclusion from the labour market' led Levitas (1996) to question whether the original European policies served to obscure and, therefore, perpetuate less visible dimensions of inequality. More specifically, Roulstone (2000) has recently argued that the way disability problems are framed within the 'New Deal' and 'Welfare to Work' have not substantially challenged excluding practices amongst employers, and risk reaffirming stereotypes of disabled people as wilfully dependent.

Another narrow channel down which the 'inclusion' debate has been allowed to trickle is inclusion in planning of health and social care services.

The new Labour Government's first specific paper on mental health, *Modernising Mental Health Services*, was subtitled *Safe, Sound and Supportive* (DoH, 1998). On the one hand, this emphasised the safety of the public as the paramount concern, while on the other, promising services more responsive to individual needs — two opposing measures in terms of 'user-empowerment'. This paper was rapidly followed by the *National Service Framework for Mental Health*, which cited the involvement of 'service users and their carers in the planning and delivery of care' as the first of ten 'guiding values and principles'. However, the content failed to expound significantly on the implications of this value. The seven 'standards' of the main document dealt at length with concerns of other stakeholders, with two standards on evidence (for academics and clinicians) and one on carers, but seemed to ignore service users (NHS, 1999).

Interested parties had to wait another eight months until the publication of the *NHS Plan* for a coherent picture of how the Government proposed to structure user-involvement (NHS, 2000). The Plan rehashed the old consumerist ideas of 'choice' and 'consultation', as well as talking about the citizenship, without addressing any of the weaknesses outlined above. The proposed patients' forums and citizenship panels take no specific account of the needs of mental health service users — a point picked out by the Health Select Committee in its report on mental health services. Also, unlike the community health councils that they are replacing, the new forums will have no 'teeth' with which to force the trusts who 'consult' with them to take notice of what they say.

On a more positive note, the Plan proposes a national patient advocacy liaison service, which will co-ordinate advocates in every hospital. This point is expanded upon in the White Paper for a new Mental Health Act, which will locate a new right to independent advocacy alongside more contentious powers for compulsory treatment in the community and the detention of people solely on the basis of risk to others. *The Guardian* (26 June, 2002) justifiably reported that the driving force behind the new mental health bill is not a concern for patients rights, but a desire to appease widespread media inspired concern over the risks that patients with mental health problems pose to the community.

Research methods and empowerment

An interesting feature of the National Service Framework was its explicit dependence on 'research evidence'. This can be seen as symptomatic of a wider movement, both nationally and internationally, towards 'evidence-based medicine' (Clarke, 1999). Interestingly, the NSF grades the methodologies into five levels: the only one mentioning service users is 'Type 5' — expert opinion. This classification completely ignores the body of emergent 'participatory', 'empowering', 'emancipatory' or 'anti-oppressive' research approaches in mental health.

There is a continued debate concerning the distinguishing characteristics of 'participatory' and 'emancipatory' research (Zarb, 1992; Troyna, 1994), and the problems with participatory evaluation (Gregory, 2000). Barnes and Wistow (1992) highlighted many of the practical and political problems associated with achieving models of user-involvement in research which are beneficial beyond the experience of having a voice.

Yeich and Levine (1992) have suggested that participatory research involves 'oppressed people in the study of and solution to social problems' (p. 1894), and that participation should result in the transformation of social structure. This is reminiscent of a 'critical' social research in its desire to challenge and change given structures (Harvey, 1990). However, the distinction can be made between the shared intent, and the adoption here of a familiar 'empowering' mode, when they consider the role of the participant in the research process. They introduce this very central issue when they add:

The idea of a researcher designing an intervention to empower other people is somewhat contradictory. Empowerment seems to be a process that one must do for oneself — not something that someone can do for or to another.

(Yeich and Levine, 1992, p. 1907)

Similarly, while Zarb (1992) does consider there to be a distinction between 'participatory' and 'emancipatory' research, he argues that for research to be truly emancipatory, it must lead to the empowerment of (disabled) people. This, he argues, can only ever be achieved by a pre-requisite level of participation, and where the control of the research process is held by the disabled people themselves. Zarb (1992) and Oliver (1992) agree that empowerment cannot be given, but is 'something that people must take for themselves'. The arguments that they pose, could equally be applied to people who have experienced discrimination and exclusion within traditional mental health service delivery, care or the research process (Faulkner and Nicholls, 1999).

Zarb (1992) realistically suggests that the current debates are set within the historical context of research methodology. Both Zarb (1992) and Oliver (1992) agree that the 'social relations of research production' have historically and inherently served to distort the representation of (disabled) people, by the technicalities of research. More specifically, these technicalities are setting the research agenda, and formulating the study design. The absence of disabled representation or involvement in this process renders the relationship as unequal and 'flawed'. Davis (1992) has also highlighted the experience of participants feeling 'used' by researchers. However, providing the right situation or relation for 'empowerment' locates the researcher quite differently from both traditional research and 'critical' research practices. Thus, in an anti-oppressive paradigm, the role of the participant is constructed as active within the research process. Davis (1992) considers 'empowerment' to be demonstrated through the participants' full and early involvement in setting the research agenda.

Here, Zarb (1992) is aware that the research community are not necessarily 'ready' for such a re-location of the 'object' as 'subject' as 'participant' or as Freire would assert 'co-investigator' (Freire, 1970 [1996]). Sohng (1992) would be more cynical, and suggests that the participant would not be 'trusted'. Zarb (1992) illustrates his concern:

> *So, at last we can begin to identify a research agenda for emancipatory disability research; not the disabled people of the positivist and interpretative research paradigms but the disablism ingrained in the individualistic consciousness and institutionalised practices of what is, ultimately, a disablist society. These are the issues that disabled people*

> *have placed on the research agenda; the key issue for the research community is whether or not they can respond.*
>
> (Zarb, 1992, p. 112)

In a challenge to the research communities, Oliver (1992) is making an explicit statement relating to the oppressive nature of research:

> *... do researchers wish to join with disabled people and use their expertise and skills in their struggles against oppression or do they wish to continue to use these skills and expertise in ways in which disabled people find oppressive?*
>
> (Oliver, 1992, p. 102)

Feminist methodology(ies) is equally concerned with the respective roles of the researcher and researched and the relationship between them (Roberts, 1981; Oakley, 1992). However, despite a general acknowledgement of the 'empowerment' of the subject within a feminist paradigm, there is considerable debate relating to the extent to which emancipatory claims are achieved (Hammersley, 1995). Troyna (1994), for example, would be critical of all research claims as emancipatory.

Acker *et al* (1991) would agree that the problems of doing emancipatory research have not, as yet, been solved and would, no doubt, agree with Oliver (1992) who argues for the development of new and alternative research methods that are compatible within an anti-oppressive framework. They are keen, however, to stress a continuing commitment to the inclusion of the researched as an active subject in the research process and suggest that the process should not become, 'only another mode of oppression'.

Following on from Oliver (1992) and Acker *et al* (1991), it is important to note that a basic principle of anti-oppressive research paradigm is to avoid the replication of 'alienating' and 'outsider' experiences of participants.

However in this context, Acker *et al* (1991) identify a specific difficulty with participation: the lack of technical knowledge which impedes equal participation. They give participatory involvement in the analysis of the data as a specific example. They attribute the basis of a wider problem to a lack of shared interest, ideology and language. It could be argued that an anti-oppressive research methodology is, in part, an extension to a (merely) 'critical' research methodology. That would be one interpretation. While the theoretical frameworks are common critique(s), it follows that there is considerable scope for differences within and between standpoints. The significant factor in relation to the overall polemic resides in its potential for praxis. Its appeal is more than a political allegiance, it is about the ability to use theory in a thoughtful and reflective capacity, and apply it to practice through 'user-led analysis and user-led action' (Ward and Mullender, 1993).

'Empowerment' towards a shared language?

McLean (1995) has argued that the concept of 'empowerment' has been 'diluted', 'distorted' and 'has assumed diverse and even contradictory, meanings'. This confusion is illustrated when Rodwell (1996) asks, 'is empowerment a process or a product?' Thus, McLean says:

> ... *It may refer to a process, a goal to be achieved, or a combination of these. It may also refer to processes occurring in relation to the individual, the organisation or the larger social structure, or to interrelations among these levels. Finally, it may be used to refer to a service approach — a radical departure from its original meaning for ex-patients concerned with self-determination and challenging professional control.*

(McLean, 1995, p. 1056)

Kieffer (1984) has also argued that the 'applicability' of empowerment, despite its theoretical and practical 'appeal', 'has been limited by continuing conceptual ambiguity'. His research study investigating individual empowerment of 'emerging grassroot activists' suggests that the process of empowerment is necessarily long-term. In constructing a framework of citizen empowerment around 'adult learning and development', Kieffer offered an alternative approach to the study of traditional explorations of empowerment, away from the focus of powerlessness and onto the search for individual meanings associated with becoming personally and socio-politically empowered.

Importantly, in a substantial critique of varying models, McLean (1995, p. 1059) offers a definition of empowerment that adds to the individual dimension of empowerment through the 'societal level, acting to transform social conditions through laws and policies that challenge discriminatory practices'. Segal *et al* (1995) have demonstrated the different outcomes associated with 'personal empowerment' and 'organisational empowerment' within American self-help agencies. Of the former, they assert a high relationship between independent social functioning, quality of life and a claimed individual empowerment. Secondly, as member participation, having an active role in the organisation, offers a dimension of 'control and influence' that they directly attribute to becoming 'empowered'.

This line of argument is important here, as it suggests that power differentials exist unchallenged between user and provider. Where it might appear that service users are actively being invited to participate under the name of 'empowerment', the structures of traditional service delivery will remain intact (Rogers, Pilgrim and Lacey, 1993).

The development of user-involvement in response to the NHS and Community Care Act 1990, has been evaluated by Bowl (1996). In researching the implementation of user involvement within the sphere of social services, Bowl examined the extent to which users were involved in decision making, the extent to which users felt valued, and the extent to which they felt empowered. He found several interesting issues: users often felt 'ill-prepared' for participation in planning or strategic-management decision making; a varying level of agreement regarding the extent to which they were taken 'seriously'; and some users who felt 'very disempowered' due to their limited knowledge and experience. He also suggests that people do not experience involvement as power-sharing due to the lack of 'participative' democracy they have previously experienced within the mental health system. This was particularly felt where they had been subject to compulsory detention.

In addition, Bowl was interested in the 'representation' and 'representativeness' of users' views. He became aware of the fundamental difficulty in securing a 'real' representation. Like others, (for example, Williams *et al*, 1996), he is alerted to this as a common source of criticism of all consumer/user-involvement initiatives. Moreover, this is an issue that is well recognised within user/activist groups (Campbell, 1996). However, while there is the push and the authority to 'involve' users, the complaints remain that the user does not truly 'represent' users; and this is used as a 'truth' claim that user-involvement cannot work. This 'truth' is never applied to each of the involved professionals — that they do not necessarily represent their particular group, but this is often taken as an *a priori* assumption.

Glenister (1994) in a review of patient participation in psychiatric services, found that theoretical frameworks for defining participation were largely inadequate, and studies undertaken did not seek the views of the participants as participants. In the same way that Oliver (1992) blames 'the alienation of disabled people from the process of research' for the failure to influence policy; many service developments within mental health are established without the real involvement of the users (Williams *et al*, 1996; Strathdee and Thornicroft, 1993; Rogers *et al*, 1993).

Similarly, the relationships inherent in health care must also be equally culpable in that the discourses embodied within the professional knowledge-base are maintained, and therefore unshared, unchallenged and possessed, in tact, by the professionals. Smith (1988) has argued that much depends on how the problem is understood by the professional. Again, we are reminded of the assumed 'superiority' of the 'expert', and should be alerted to the forbearance that is disguised behind the 'implementation' of patient participation. Schafer (1996), amongst others, reminds us that mental health professionals are seen by users of the service, to be part of the problem and not the solution. Bowl's identification of 'professional over-rule' demonstrates a tension between inviting 'participation' or 'involvement', and maintaining restrictive practices (Bowl, 1996). A clear distinction should be made between the politics of 'participation' or 'involvement'and 'empowerment'. These concepts are often used interchangeably, yet as constructions they are quite different in the level of involvement and control that is 'given' (like a gift?) to the user and importantly, the 'transfer of power' (Bowl, 1996).

Conclusion

In conclusion of this discussion, it would seem apparent that the discourse of 'empowerment' within the public domain is highly complex. At a basic level, there is disparity in the terminology relating to the involvement of service users. This may, or may not, reflect the underlying ideologies and varying (party) political intentions that either include or exclude individual or community participation in decision making (Croft and Beresford, 1992). The level of control and influence that is achieved in the name of empowerment will continue to rely heavily on the willingness of authorities and 'legitimate' holders of power or authority to engage genuinely in the debate. Moreover, where this term 'empowerment' is frequently used to illustrate (false) developments within mental health, it would be naive to conclude that the 'authorities' and professionals have conceded a pre-existing 'oppression(s)'.

Consequently, a range of difficulties are posed for the development of an effective and consistent strategy of 'empowerment'. A meaningful response to this would perhaps seek to fuse a critical approach, which is fundamentally cognisant of the 'oppression(s)' and power issues apparent within the structures and relations of psychiatric and mental healthcare practice; with a demonstrable empowering approach. We would argue that parallels exist within the difficulties of empowerment at the levels of individual citizenship, and the power to change agenda at a social and political level. Where policy and research have traditionally subjugated the service user within both structures and processes, there is a paradoxical shift towards 'inclusion' or 'involvement'. While this shift might lie in the language of current policy, we would argue that it remains a potential while the power and resources in mental health policy and research largely remain intact.

Key points

- ✻ 'User involvement' may be perceived as desirable from consumerist, medical, citizenship, academic or service users own (political) perspectives. Margaret Thatcher's commitment to a consumerist and market driven healthcare system paved the way for increased user participation.

- ✻ Many Government reports which have purported to promote user involvement have proved to be rhetoric.

- ✻ Participation may be driven from a shared feeling of disenfranchisement and powerlessness together with an individual and collective demand for choices, self-determination and control.

- ✻ Successive Government papers have identified the notion of citizenship as being important to their success, however, they are limited in their actual engagement of citizens and often completely neglect the users of mental health services.

- ✻ There is a place for participation and emancipatory research and service users have a great deal to offer the evidence base.

References

Acker J (1991) Hierarchies, jobs, bodies: A theory of gendered organisations. In: Lorber J, Farrell SA, eds. *The Social Construction of Gender*. Sage, Newbury Park, CA: 162–79

Barnes M, Wistow G, eds (1992) *Researching User Involvement*. Nuffield Institute Seminar Series

Bowl R (1996) Legislating For User Involvement in the UK: Mental Health Services And The NHS and Community Care Act. *Int J Soc Psychiatry* **42**(3): 165–80

Campbell P (1996) The history of the user movement in the United Kingdom. In Heller T, Reynolds J, Gomm R, Muston R, Pattison S, eds (1996) *Mental Health Matters*. Macmillan Press Ltd, Basingstoke

Clarke MJ, Stewart LA (1997) Meta-analyses using individual patient data. *J Eval Clin Pract* **3**(3): 207–12

Clarke JB (1999) Evidence-based practice: a retrograde step? The importance of pluralism in evidence generation for the practice of health care. *J Clin Nurs* **8**(1): 89–94

Crane S (1998) *Shrink Resistant: The Survivor Movement and the Survivor Perspective*. US Network, Aberystwyth

Croft S, Beresford P (1992) The politics of participation. *Critical Social Policy***12**(2): 20–44

Davis CA (1992) The effects of music and basic relaxation instruction on pain and anxiety of women undergoing in-office gynecological procedures. *J Music Therapy* **29**(4): 202–18

Department of Health (1998) *Modernising mental health services: safe, sound and supportive*. DoH, London

Faulkner A, Nicholls V (1999) Strategies for Living. *Mental Health Care* **3**(1): 28–29

Forbes J, Sashidharan P (1997) User involvement in services — incorporation or challenge? *Br J Social Work* **27**: 481–98

Freire P (1970) *Pedagogy of the Oppressed*. Translated by Myra Bergman Ramos, 1921. Penguin, London, revised edition 1970

Glenister D (1994) Patient participation in psychiatric services: a literature review and proposal for a research strategy. *J Adv Nurs* **19**: 802–11

Grace VM (1991) The marketing of empowerment and the construction of the health consumer : a critique of health promotion. *Int J Health Services* **21**(2): 329–43

Green D (1990) *The NHS Reforms: whatever happened to consumer choice?* Institute of Economic Affairs, London

Gregory A (2000) *Problematizing Participation*, Evaluation 6 (2). Sage Publications: 179–99

Hammersley M (1995) *The Politics of Social Research*. Sage, London

Harvey L (1990) *Critical Social Research*. Unwin Hyman, GB

Hickson DJ, McCullough AF (1980) Power in organizations. In: Salaman G, Thompson K, eds. *Control and Ideology in Organizations*. MIT Press, Cambridge, Mass

Kieffer CH (1984) Citizen empowerment: a developmental perspective. *Prevention in Human Services* **3**: 201–26

Levitas R (1996) The concept of social exclusion and the new Durkheimian Hegemony. *Critical Social Policy* **46**(16): 5–20

Lindow V, Morris J (1995) *Service user involvement: Synthesis of findings and experience in the field of community care*. Joseph Rountree Foundation, York

McLean A (1995) Empowerment and the psychiatric consumer/ex-patient movement in The United States: contradictions, crisis and change. *Soc Sci Med* **40**(8): 1053–71

Mullender A, Ward D (1985) Towards an alternative model of social groupwork. *Br J Social Work* **15**: 155–72

National Health Service (1999) *A first class service: quality in the new NHS: feedback on consultations*. NHS Executive, London

National Health Service (2000) *The NHS Plan: a plan for investment, a plan for reform*. DoH, London

Nettleton S (1995) *The Sociology of Health and Illness*. Polity Press, Cambridge

Oakley A (1992) *Taking it like a woman*. Flamingo, London

Oliver M (1992) Changing the social relations of research production? *Disability, Handicap & Society*, **7**(2)

Opie A (1992) Qualitative research, appropriation of the 'other' and empowerment. *Feminist Review* **40**, Spring: 52–69

Parsons T (1951) *The Social System*. The Free Press, Glencoe

Paton C (1990) *The Prime Minister's Review of the National Health Service and the 1989 White Paper Working For Patients*. DoH, London

Paton C (1998) *Competition and Planning in the NHS: The Consequences of the NHS Reforms*. Stanley Thornes (Publishers) Limited, London

Rhodes P, Nocon A (1998) User Involvement and the NHS Reforms. *Health Expectations* **1**: 73–81

Roberts H (1981) *Doing Feminist Research*. Flamingo, London

Rodwell CM (1996) An analysis of the concept of empowerment. *J Adv Nurs* **23**: 305–13

Rogers A, Pilgrim D, Lacey R (1993) *Experiencing Psychiatry — Users' views of Services*. Macmillan Press Ltd, Hong Kong

Roulstone A (2000) Disability, dependency and the new deal for disabled people. *Disability and Society* **15**(3): 427za–43

Schafer T (1996) Empowering service users; the myth, the reality and the hope. *J Psychiatric Mental Health Nurs* **3**: 391–4

Sedgewick P (1982) *Psychopolitics*. Pluto Press, London

Segal ZV, Gemar M, Truchon C, Guirguis M, Horowitz LM (1995) A priming methodology for studying self-representation in major depressive disorder. *J Abnorm Psychol* **104**(1): 205–13

Smith R (1988) The halo effect. *Nurs Times* **84**(51): 68

Sohng S (1992) Consumers as research partners. *J Progressive Human Services* **3**(2): 1–14

Strathdee G, Thornicroft G (1993) Social consequences. In: Bhugra D, Leff J, eds. *Principles of Social Psychiatry*. Blackwell Scientific Publications, Oxford

Troyna B (1994) Blind faith? Empowerment and educational research. *Int Stud Sociology of Education* **4**(1): 3–24

Ward D, Mullender A (1993) Empowerment and oppression: an indissoluble pairing for contemporary social work. In: Walmsley J, Reynolds J, Shakespeare P, Woolfe R, eds. *Health, Welfare and Practice*. Sage Publications, London: 147–53

Williams R, Emerson G, Muth Z, eds (1996) *Voices in partnership — involving users and carers in commissioning and delivering mental health services*. NHS Health Advisory Service, Location?

Yeich S, Levine R (1992) Participatory research's contribution to the conceptualization of empowerment. *J Applied Soc Psychol* **22**(24): 1894–1908

Zarb G (1992) On the road to Damascus: first steps towards changing the relations of disability research production. *Disability, Handicap & Society* **7**(2)

3

Patient and public participation in health systems: some basic principles

Bob Sang

Advocacy and the roots of participation

Over twenty years ago, in the period immediately following the long-stay hospital scandals of the late 1970s, I was involved in establishing the United Kingdom's first **independent** citizen advocacy schemes (Sang and O'Brien, 1984). Since that time, it is no accident that we have seen a considerable growth — both in advocacy schemes and in the movement of patients' organisations (Sang, 1999). But it is only recently within this twenty-year evolution that public authorities have begun to address the issue of patient and public participation in health systems, by identifying ways and means of engaging with lay people that supplemented traditional, formal duties to consult. From the 'Local Voices' initiative of the early 1990s to the latest circular instructions, successive governments have endeavoured to encourage and direct NHS organisations to achieve greater 'patient and public participation' in the NHS. But, what does this mean? What is the purpose — or, are the purposes? And, how will we know effective and appropriate 'participation' when we see it?

I want to revisit these questions in this contribution and to offer an analysis that confronts many of the current assumptions about 'patient and public participation'. In so doing, I shall address the risk that we achieve no more than the consolidation of ad hoc, reactive responses to ill thought-out policy and thereby, only a partial understanding of the challenges of creating genuinely participatory health systems.

I shall begin by addressing some of the more uncomfortable and distressing aspects of our health and care systems.

I had become involved in independent lay advocacy because, after over ten years' experience of our 'caring' services, where I had observed both inspiring professionalism and chronic abuse in equal measure (and everything in between), I wanted to test the simple idea that '**patients**' could really be at the centre of the development and improvement of services.

When 'blowing the whistle' on abuse, I had found myself, more often than not aligned with the victims: children in care, elderly hospital patients, people with learning difficulties. As other whistle-blowers have found, abuse (often the persistent demeaning of individuals and not just the overt physical and sexual attacks about which the public learn from time to time) is marginalised as 'exceptional', or even 'a misunderstanding'. The 'whistleblower', herself or himself, becomes defined as the problem, risking their career and even, on occasions, their personal safety (Beardshaw, 1981).

Despite the dark, abusive, side of working in human services, I had learned also that when individuals — from young children to very frail elders — feel safe, and when they feel supported and valued as fellow citizens, they begin to share their thoughts and feelings, their experiences and aspirations, in uncluttered and mature ways. For example, when I helped to facilitate one of the early 'Who Cares' groups for children in care, initiated by the National Children's Bureau in the mid-1970s, the children themselves articulated very clear and sensible views about improving their care. They also knew where the abusers were in the system.

Our 'Who Cares' group' used a local, independently funded community centre, and the children (aged from five to fifteen) raised their own funding to cover costs. These 'vulnerable', 'at risk' young people showed great insight into their own circumstances, a realistic assessment of their prospects, and great frustration with the authorities and professionals who never appeared to listen to them. They taught us that everyone can have a **voice** and, if that voice is not heard, then we have little chance of developing appropriate and sensitive services. Twenty-five years on, we now have cumulative and distressing evidence of the systematic failure of our childcare systems — systems where abuse became endemic within some services. Yet, 'Who Cares' remains a relatively marginalised network, and thousands of children are never heard, never valued as younger fellow citizens, capable of contributing to better services and better lives, in the longer run.

In the early 1980s, such oppressive circumstances existed systemically for tens of thousands of adults: disabled people, 'mentally handicapped' people, psychiatric patients, and elderly people living in institutions. As within childcare, countless reports accumulated (Martin with Evans, 1984), and the original Green Paper on Community Care was published (Department of Health and Social Security, 1981).

The then Government recognised the potential of citizen advocacy, as one means of supporting the large numbers of individuals who had no voice, by contributing to the first project founded by five national charities (Sang and O'Brien, 1984). Citizen advocacy is a simple idea: an ordinary citizen befriends and supports someone who has no voice — for example, a profoundly disabled person — ensuring that he/she achieves their rights as citizens and a reasonable quality of life. Thousands of citizen advocacy relationships have developed in the last twenty years (Citizen Advocacy Information and Training, 1998), as has the independent self-advocacy movement (see below), and more recently the 'expert patient' movement, which builds on the principles of self-management. But, before I reflect on the learning of such direct participation in health systems, it is worth highlighting the two critical lessons learned from the early developments of independent lay advocacy, for they apply to all aspects of modern health systems. After all, we all have the potential to become vulnerable and voiceless at some time in our lives.

First and foremost, everyone can have a voice, no matter how ill or disabled they are. Many of the people I met in long-stay institutions in the 1980s had been isolated and institutionalised for up to fifty years. Fifty years of abandonment; no family or friends to visit them and monitor their circumstances. They were entirely dependent on paid staff for their care and well-being. Remember, these fellow citizens of ours were not compulsorily detained, they were 'voluntary' patients or residents: just as anyone might be who enters a hospital or a nursing home following an accident or illness. In **every** patient case, three kinds of decision should be considered:

- admission and discharge, whereby people 'negotiate' their terms of engagement with the health system
- consent to treatment, the informed and shared responsibility for specific interventions proposed for direct users of a health system; and more controversially
- planning decisions that can affect the lives of individuals, groups and even whole communities.

In the 1980s, we rediscovered what happens when these decisions were not considered, and when their quality and reliability were taken for granted, especially when 'patients', our fellow citizens, had no voice.

Two examples will suffice.

Mary lived in a 'villa' with ten other women in the grounds of a large institution. Mary had cerebral palsy and had been institutionalised from a very early age. In her mid-twenties she was 'mothered' by her housemates, all in their sixties and seventies; 'moral defectives' who had been compulsorily detained under the pre-war Mental Deficiency

Acts. Mary was defined as 'non-verbal' because, as far as hospital staff were concerned, she could speak very few words. Her citizen advocate, Ann, a local teacher, soon discovered that Mary was articulate and socially skilled when away from the institution. I became involved when Ann rang me to ask for my support because Mary, who had been growing in confidence, had been placed, sedated, in a locked ward away from the villa. Unbeknown to us, a planning decision had been taken to close Mary's villa and when staff came to move her, she had become very distressed. Years before she had been prescribed Largactil, the 'liquid cosh' so, on reviewing her notes, the duty doctor had relied on the same remedy. Ann and I found a subdued, tearful Mary in bed in a crowded ward – quite a contrast from her own room in the relatively secluded villa she shared with her friends. When I asked the hospital manager about the decision to close the villa and the consequent events, it became clear that neither he nor the medical team perceived any reason for involving Mary or Ann in the decision-making process or in the subsequent treatment and incarceration decisions. And, at the time, there were no accessible, independent means of redress. Mary now lives happily in supported housing with housemates of her own choosing. It has been a long and ultimately, worthwhile journey.

The issues of accountability and decision making without reference to the actual patient concerned, highlighted in Mary's story, apply also within the so-called 'acute' hospital sector as my second example shows.

Norman's GP admitted his seventy-two-year-old patient to the local hospital trust because a persistent chest infection was worsening, with a risk of pneumonia. It was a routine admission and Norman's return was anticipated within a few days. The GP had kept Norman's sister informed and everyone was happy with the decision to admit Norman to hospital. Within hours, Norman was dead and the hospital authorities claimed his death was a result of a rapid worsening in his condition. Unhappy with this explanation, Norman's sister persisted with her enquiries and it took two arduous years to establish the facts. At the final formal Complaints hearing, his sister's worst fears were confirmed: Norman had not been properly admitted or cared for, and had choked to death alone and unsupervised in a side ward.

Norman's sister died the day after the hearing. Getting to that point had cost her so much, and worse was to follow. The health authorities refused to follow up the recommendations of that hearing and ensure that service improvements were implemented: it was only when her family went to the national press with the story that things changed. It is fair to say that the radical improvement that subsequently took place at the hospital resulted from exceptional professional leadership, and a real willingness to learn the lessons from this tragic case, but only after a total of four years' persistence by Norman's family.

Sadly, the NHS complaints system remains relatively inaccessible and trapped within the structures of the service itself, and the need for independent lay advocacy has never been greater (Sang and Clements, 2000). Independent, contestable means of redress are still not readily available to patients and their families and friends (Public Law Report, 1999). This is just not acceptable in a society of increasing diversity, where we will have to create systems that are open and responsive to people of all ages, abilities, and cultures.

In the next section, I shall examine the lessons we can learn from recent attempts to engage with patients and the public, across the NHS and the wider care system. But, bluntly, all this work is mere froth if ordinary people are not afforded accessible and contestable, independently managed, means of redress. Nor is it worth the candle if the voice of individuals is not supported and heard 'at every level in every process' (Sang, 1998).

Everyone involved in Mary and Norman's case would have gained, without the appalling distress that was actually caused, if their voice had been heard. Ultimately, in a genuinely participatory system, it is the individual end-users (patients, clients, carers, etc., whatever the label) who must be the drivers of positive change and the initiators of learning. The health system is still 'stood on its head', serving the interests of internal groups and authorities. Can it be stood on its feet? As a former Chief Medical Officer recently noted: 'We are calling for a paradigm shift... but it will only be a paradigm shift if it is patient-led.' (Donaldson, 2000).

Unpacking participation: whose system is it anyway?

I was recently asked to respond to a research tender concerned with 'eliciting the views of patients'. It seemed very rational and timely: a literature study, including the Internet, followed by a scoping exercise to determine the extent of the use of the emerging typology of methods. As I read through the well-intentioned specification, I became increasingly angry. Had these academics and NHS researchers learned nothing and understood less? Why waste public money on a redundant exercise? Did they not realise that 'we' had moved well beyond this traditional research paradigm? Let me explain the sources of my ire.

Consider what it is really like to engage with a system that depends on labelling its principal participants ('patient', 'client', 'handicapped', 'the fractured hip in bed 3') and researching them as if they were supermarket customers — research that confirms and even deepens the culture of dependency sustaining contemporary health systems. From highly selective, risk averse, private health insurance schemes; through an institutionalising independent sector of care; to monolithic public service provision, we have built a system that presumes the dependence of whole populations on the 'expertise' and hierarchical structures that constitute the largely unaccountable bureaucracies dominating our health provision (Priestley, 1999). People are cast in the role of '**victim**'— passive, uninformed patient with cancer, or depression, or Down's syndrome. And, victims beget heroes: the professionals, managers and politicians to come to rescue them in their time of need. This psychopathology of care is deeply embedded in the self-esteem and career interests of those who work in our caring services. It is rarely challenged, and even when things go badly wrong, as in the recent Ledward and Shipman cases, such dangerous doctors proclaim themselves victims of a flawed system!

It is well established that in any human system where power is distributed heavily in favour of one group or groups, then the risks to the least powerful groups grow (Goffman, 1968). All talk of 'patient involvement' in modernising our health services is misleading and meaningless while we fail to address these issues of power and psychological damage in our health systems. Fortunately, a number of forces are at work that make this much more possible. They fall into two categories: independent, patient-led development; and, enabling policy contexts. For example:

❖ Patient-led research and development is proliferating, facilitated by the Standing Advisory Group on consumer involvement in NHS research (NHS Executive, 1999).

❖ The disability and 'expert patient' movements, led in health care by the Long-term Medical Conditions Alliance (LMCA), have demonstrated how much people with chronic conditions can take charge of their own lives and work in mature, co-operative relationships with clinical teams and multi-agency services.

❖ Independent lay advocacy schemes have grown in number and accessibility, focusing on ensuring that the voices of our most vulnerable fellow citizens are heard in respect of all the decisions that affect their lives (Clements and Sang, 2000).

❖ The College of Health, working with services users and carers, has developed training materials aimed specifically at patients who will act as members of decision-making bodies in health (Fletcher and Bradburn, 1999).

❖ Finally, we now know that through such means as citizens' juries, lay people can take on and resolve tough health policy and planning decisions (Elizabeth, 1999).

All of this grounded participatory work will be of little value if the organisations and institutions of our wider health system do not themselves become more open and responsive. Until now, they have relied on deploying a range of methods (Chambers, 2000) without shifting the structural and cultural assumptions that underlie their functions and use of resources. However, as Governments and some leading thinkers endeavour to unlock our health systems, a mix of consumerist and communitarian principles and practices have been deployed in an attempt to unfreeze our health and care bureaucracies. Can this emerging alignment of policy and patient empowerment help us to create genuinely participatory health systems, despite the considerable vested interests and deep pathology of expert dependency that stand in the way?

Recognising that we have yet to guarantee patients and the public independently supported means of achieving a voice, or even access to fair means of redress in our system, as it stands today, the following model (*Figure 3.1*) attempts to clarify the essence of the challenge we face.

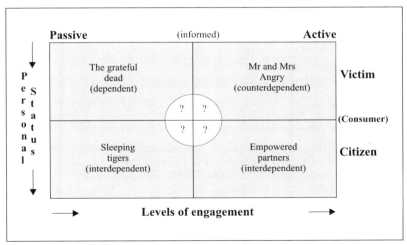

Figure 3.1: Towards lay participation in health systems

How can we take advantage of the new consumerism — middle-class voter driven though it may be — to achieve a more sustainable partnership for health and care? This is the goal of patient and public involvement work. This contribution builds on the principles established above, and recognises that **'we'** — patients and the public — have a responsibility as active, informed citizens to 'break' the dependency culture which fuels the institutions and bureaucracies of the health sector.

Key points

- Although advocacy schemes were established in the UK over twenty years ago, it is only recently that statutory services have started to consider seriously service user and public participation in health services.

- Potentially, all service users and carers can 'have a voice', but in practice, they are often ignored, as are professional 'whistle-blowers', who have often been penalised for their efforts.

- The 'Who Cares' groups established that children in care were able to put forward valuable views on improving their care. There have been considerable developments in self-advocacy and citizen advocacy in the last two decades. There is a need for readily available redress; and lay advocacy in relation to complaints, particularly as NHS complaints systems are 'relatively inaccessible.'

- When professionals and managers fail to consider the views of service users and carers, or involve them in decision making, serious problems result. These include adverse effects on service users' care and quality of life. This is illustrated with reference to problems faced by two individuals, who lacked opportunities for their voice to be heard.

- Many health services label service users and place them in 'victim' roles. Discussions about service user participation are meaningless unless issues concerning power, and the psychological damage experienced by some service users, are addressed.

- Recently, various local and national initiatives and Central Government policies have enabled increases in service user and carer empowerment, participation and advocacy. However, the value of such initiatives will be limited unless health services 'become more open and responsive.'

- A model of service user/citizen participation in health services is presented. The model includes different levels of engagement and personal status.

References

Beardshaw V (1989) *Nurse Whistleblowers at Work.* Social Audit, London

Chambers R (2000) *Involving Patients and the Public.* Radcliffe Medical Press, Abingdon

Citizen Advocacy Information and Training (1998) *Standing By Me.* Citizen Advocacy Information, London

Clements J, Sang B (2000) Voices of difference. *J Medical Law*

Department of Health and Social Security (1981) *Care in the Community. A Consultative Document on Moving Resources for Care in England.* DHSS, London: July

Donaldson L (2000) Introductory remarks to the 'Expert Patient' Conference, London, July

Elizabeth S (1999) *Ordinary Wisdom.* King's Fund, London

Fletcher G, Bradburn J (1999) *Voices in Action.* College of Health, London

Goffman, E. (1968) *Asylums: Essays on the social situations of patients and other inmates.* Penguin Books, Harmondsworth

Martin J with Evans D (1984) *Hospitals in Trouble. Robertson, Oxford*

NHS Executive (1999) *Involvement Works.* Department of Health, London: April

Priestley M (1999) *Disability, Politics and Community Care.* Jessica Kingsley, London

Sang B, O'Brien J (1984) *Advocacy.* King's Fund, London

Sang B (1998) *A Second Better Chance. Report on the Future of the NHS to the NHS.* 50th Anniversary Conference. King's Fund, London

Sang B (1999) The customer is sometimes right. *Health Services Journal*: August

Sang B, Clements J (2000) Voices of difference. *J Medical Law*

Sang B, O'Brien J (1984) *Advocacy.* King's Fund, London

4

Giving birth to participation. Are women empowered within the maternity services?

Nessa McHugh

What is informed choice? What is a free informed choice? How free, how well informed must an act be to deserve the name of choice, as opposed to unthinking imitation of others, or, indeed, doing the only thing that circumstances allow?

(Reid, 1992, p. 3)

Our vision is that each woman is treated as an individual. She is given all the information she needs to decide what type of care is most appropriate for her and her baby. The woman is supported in her choice, whatever it might be.

(Maternity Action in Leicestershire, 1996, p. 1)

Introduction

Childbirth and motherhood are pivotal features of many women's lives, regardless of ethnicity, class or background. The decisions to have children, not to have children, or to delay parenthood are all features of contemporary British society. Difficulty in conception involves decisions around the infertility process previously unavailable. Women are assumed to be in control of their fertility to a level previously unobtainable. Even if those assumptions do not reflect the reality of all women's lives, which often they do not, pregnancy and childbirth are still seen as normal physiological states (at least, that's the rhetoric of the childbirth campaigners). The majority of women will progress through pregnancy and birth in a state of health and well-being. For many women pregnancy may be the first time they have any prolonged contact with health services, and going into hospital to give birth may be the first time that a woman has stayed in a hospital. Pregnancy and birth may also potentially represent the first real experience of health services as something other than a benevolent public service. When a woman's expectations of childbirth are not met it undermines and detracts from the experience.

> *I found that the staff were very busy and I was just left to get on with it (breastfeeding her baby). In the end I just went and got a bottle off the trolley, it seemed much easier. I couldn't wait to get home, the ward was dirty, I didn't dare have a bath, it was noisy and forget trying to have any rest. It was just the pits.*

(A twenty-nine-year-old woman's account of her first stay in hospital following the birth of her daughter)

Ethnicity, class and background will without doubt effect the expectations of a woman and her family group, and the nature of interaction between the pregnant woman and the service providers. Social class and ethnicity are factors that directly influence the type of care that women are likely to receive, in terms of information, choice and intervention.

> *This is particularly important (informed choice) if the women have different cultural expectations from those of the doctors, midwives, nurses and other health professionals in charge. Unless the flexibility that has been introduced as a result of the greater choice can accommodate the different choices that women from ethnic minorities may make, the whole process of childbirth will continue to be as rigid and alienating for them as it once was for all women.*

(Commission for Racial Equality, 1994, p. 9)

This is particularly relevant when we consider that in 1995 the Clinical Standards Advisory Group found that Asian women are three times as likely to receive an episiotomy as white women. There is no physiological basis for this figure.

For some women, pregnancy and birth are characterised by confrontation and conflict, especially where the expectations of the woman are in direct conflict with the beliefs or expectations of the professionals involved with that woman's maternity care. Here, inaccuracy of information or withholding of information can be combined with emotional blackmail and scaremongering tactics to undermine the woman's confidence in herself and the choices she has made. Such approaches to care also smack of paternalism and control, despite the modern rhetoric of empowerment.

> *During my first antenatal visit to my midwife, I said I intended to have my baby at home, she informed me that I would have to see the consultant in the hospital to make that decision. She then went on to tell me that did I realise that it would hurt more at home and that I was putting my baby at risk – 'you people are all the same'.*

(Extract from the account of her first birth Judith, 1998)

Looking back

The last thirty years within the maternity services has seen a dramatic shift in the rhetoric concerning women's involvement with the planning and implementation of the maternity service provision. In 1993, the publication of *Changing Childbirth* (DoH) set out Government policy towards childbirth. For many childbirth campaigners, such as the Association for the Improvement in the Maternity Services (AIMS) and the National Childbirth Trust (NCT), this represented the culmination of years of hard campaigning to ensure that women had their voices heard in the debates surrounding the provision of appropriate care. Nationally, there was a determination to try and affect the development of services and alter attitudes and practices that are based upon tradition rather than evidence and good practice.

It could be argued that the changes in maternity provision and the increasing resistance of women to the type of service they were/are receiving mirrors the changes in women's social expectations brought about by the influence of the feminist movement in the late twentieth century. Both AIMS and the NCT had strong links with the ethos of the early feminist movement and maintain links today with the Association of Radical Midwives (ARM), another woman-focused birth movement born out of the feminist response to the increasingly medicalised arena of birth. Sheahan (1972) maintained that a state of enforced powerlessness subliminally corrupts our perceptions of ourselves leading to subordination, alienation and weakened disaffection. The increased activism of the feminist movement within the childbirth arena managed to significantly overturn the status quo to enable women to recognise the alienation experienced and turn it into a potentially powerful force for change.

Natural childbirth advocates, consumer rights activists and many feminists are united in their resistance to biomedical imperialism in childbirth and its appropriation of the power of childbearing women over their birthing experiences.

(Zadorosnzj, 1999, p.269)

This change has its basis in the ongoing determination of user organisations over the past decades to try and stem the tide of intervention and medicalisation, which characterises contemporary birth experiences for the majority of women in Britain. Oakley (1986) argued that the development of a new consumer's movement within midwifery and obstetrics heralded a historical response to the medical surveillance of pregnancy. The growth and rhetoric of consumerism within the field of childbirth suggested some level of dissonance between providers of care, policy makers and the social group, ie. women, on the receiving end of policies and care provision. Consumer groups such as the NCT were actively surveying their membership and using the information gained to try and change the quality of maternity care received by women. Information was gathered and presented in such a manner as to make it impossible to refute the truth in the assertions of consumer groups that the service was impersonal, demoralising and inappropriate.

More than half the reports carried requests for obstetricians to be 'polite', 'tactful', 'considerate', 'human not patronising', 'compassionate', 'caring'... 'truthful' and to behave with 'good manners', 'kindness' and 'thoughtfulness'. This was not because these were the qualities women had admired in their obstetricians. They are the qualities they had perceived to be lacking.

(National Childbirth Trust, 1990, p.5)

Hardey (1999) maintains that one of the dominant themes of the contemporary health arena is the proletarianisation of healthcare provision. Here changes in organisation, management and philosophy have divested professions of the control they once maintained. This is reflected in the wide range of Government reports geared to increase client participation in decision making, eg. the *Patient's Charter* (DoH, 1991), *Changing Childbirth* (DoH, 1993), *The NHS Plan* (NHS Executive, 1997), and *A First Class Service* (Audit Commission, 1997). However, many consumer groups and allied professionals would find it hard to see where exactly the medical profession has been divested of its power. Government agendas change and new health policy comes in but the medicalisation of childbirth marches on regardless of proletarianisation or any other current social phenomenon.

The NCT reported in 1994 on the availability of the *Maternity Services Charter*, the leaflet that explains women's rights and choices under the *Patient's Charter*. They found the leaflet on display in just forty-one out of 271 clinics. Of those clinics, staff at 109 maintained that they did not know about the Charter's existence. It can only be assumed that as the staff in the surveyed clinics were unaware of the charter, they were also unaware of the rights contained within them.

Focusing on the present

Changing Childbirth represented a cornerstone in the history of maternity care. It appeared that at last the views of women were being taken into account. The health professionals were left with five years to achieve the ten key recommendations (*Figure 4.1*). Changing Childbirth User forums were established around the country to help the dissemination of best practice initiatives and maintain the momentum. Maternity Service Liaison Committees, which had been technically in operation since 1984, were increased and made more effective. Generally, there was an air of optimism for the first time in many years. Seven years on it seems that only the times have changed. With a new Government and a new agenda, the aims of *Changing Childbirth* have arguably been submerged beneath other pressing health issues. The air of optimism appears to have been lost long ago and it is unclear how many of its recommendations were achieved nationally.

Where does this leave childbearing women? Are they served by health improvement programmes, health action zones, primary care trusts, midwifery-led initiatives or are they still struggling to make their voices heard in an increasingly complex health arena?

Within five years:	
1.	All women should be entitled to carry their own notes.
2.	Every woman should know one midwife who ensures continuity of her midwifery care — the named midwife.
3.	At least 30% of women should have the midwife as the lead professional.
4.	Every woman should know the lead professional who has a key role in the planning and provision of her care.
5.	At least 75% of women should know the person who cares for them during their delivery.
6.	Midwives should have direct access to some beds in all maternity units.
7.	At least 30% of women delivered in a maternity unit should be admitted under the management of a midwife.
8.	The total number of antenatal visits for women with uncomplicated pregnancies should be reviewed in the light of the available evidence and the RCOG guidelines.
9.	All front line ambulances should have a paramedic able to support the midwife who needs to transfer a woman to hospital in an emergency.
10.	All women should have access to information about the services available to them in their locality.

Figure 4.1: Indicators of success for *Changing Childbirth* (DoH, 1993, *Changing Childbirth: Report of the Expert Maternity Group*)

For many women the experience of childbirth does not appear to have been radically altered by the host of initiatives already mentioned, and choices for birth seem to be determined at a local level rather than at a national level. Childbirth pressure groups indicate that women still want a personalised service, where they can get to know the professionals providing their care (McCourt and Page, 1996), and for some women this has been achieved:

I feel that throughout this pregnancy and birth, I participated in the decisions and that I could trust my midwife. I was desperate not to have to go through a similar experience to the birth of Deborah (first baby). With Deborah, I felt very isolated. I never really got to know one midwife particularly well antenatally. The midwife who delivered Deborah was very abrupt, I had never met her before and I'm glad to say I never met her again! Looking back, I think that I was not the only woman she had to look after that day, but that was no use to me, at the time I needed someone there for me. With Kirsty, I was on a different scheme, the midwife used to come to my house and I got to know her really well. It was lovely to know that wherever I had my baby she would be there for me. So different from before and it was good to have the same midwife look after me postnatally. She became more of a friend to me really.

(Extract from Fran's account of her second birth
with a midwifery group practice scheme)

Around the country midwives and childbirth activists have been struggling to establish schemes where midwives have direct responsibility for a caseload of women. Where such schemes have become established such as BUMPS in Leicester (Birth under Midwifery Practice Scheme), they are positively evaluated in satisfaction ratings by the women concerned (Walker, 1999). These schemes are relatively small scale and the majority of women are served by the hospital systems, which remain impersonal and highly medicalised.

In the nearly eleven years since 'Changing Childbirth' was published maternity care has, sadly, not moved towards the ideals embodied in the report. Indeed, and I say this with some regret, for most women the likelihood of a normal birth with a known midwife is even less now. The centralisation and medicalisation of birth in large obstetric units has intensified rather than declined. Caesarean section rates since 'Changing Childbirth' have increased to over thirty per cent in some hospitals and have recently shown signs of rising still further.

(Winterton, 2000, p. 2)

Two questions emerge at this point: where does this leave the needs of the women who utilise the maternity services? Would it be possible to argue that actually the majority of women are perfectly content with their birth experiences and the care they receive and that it is just a vocal minority who are making excessive demands of the services?

In answer to these two questions, the audit commission report on the maternity services appeared to indicate that 90% of women were pleased with the care that they received (Audit Commission, 1997). This would seem to indicate that although the Government backed reforms of *Changing Childbirth* were largely unmet by many maternity service providers, women were getting a better service than the one campaigned against in the seventies and eighties. Yvette Cooper, Parliamentary under-Secretary for Health in the same Commons debate maintained that huge advances had been made over the past few years and that it was now safer than ever to give birth with real progress made towards a woman-centred maternity service (2000). How this rising level of safety was balanced against an increasing Caesarean section rate was not reported.

The audit report also indicated that a significant minority of women felt isolated in early labour in hospitals and that the postnatal care provided was far from satisfactory (Audit Commission, 1997).

Childbirth might possibly be perceived as safer; certainly less women die in childbirth than fifty years ago and we have health and social advantages far in excess of many countries around the world. This does not necessarily mean that women are happy with the care that they receive in Britain; they may be just relieved that the ordeal is over, and aware that elsewhere it is probably much worse? However, can relief and acceptance be seen as the same thing as active participation and ownership? Arguably not.

One of the claims made against client pressure groups within the maternity services is that they represent a vocal minority of middle-class women and the issues that they rally against are not representative of the issues that would concern all maternity service clients across the board. Green *et al* (1990) explored some of the stereotypes that surrounded pregnant women. These can loosely be defined as the over controlling 'NCT' type who were concerned with the emotional fulfilment of birth as an experience; and the 'under educated working class' woman who just wanted to get on with it. What Green *et al* revealed, was that professionals did put women into loose stereotypical categories and tended to treat women accordingly. This meant that less articulate or less educated women experienced less involvement in the decision-making process concerning their births. However, Green *et al* also found that women in this category wanted to be involved with the decisions surrounding their births and pregnancies but had lower expectations of gaining that involvement. Bluff and Holloway (1994) identified that, although many women did want to be consulted about the type of care they received, they did not always know how to communicate their needs. It would be possible to argue that based upon the conclusions drawn by Green *et al*, and Bluff and Holloway, that women have to mediate their way through service provision and the professionals are the gatekeepers of that care. Thus, things have not necessarily improved for those women who are alienated by the system on the grounds of class or ethnicity, and if the vocal minority are also not convinced that the system has improved, then whom is the system serving? It certainly does not appear to be the midwives who are also vocal in their complaints against a system that leaves them de-skilled and demoralised.

> *One of the effects of 'Changing Childbirth' has been that everyone is really nice to women and now they are 'consenting' to even more interventions. To the extent that the obscene levels of unnecessary interventions are justified on the grounds of 'women's choice'.*

> (Lawrence Beech, 2000, p. 5)

Perhaps the main driving force of client involvement in service provision has been to ensure that we manipulate women in a nicer tone of voice? Perhaps the birth environment with all its accompanying undercurrents of control has remained exactly the same; we just have pretty borders and wallpaper to hide the truth about birth politics. It is possible to argue that women still retain very little control over their birth and that birth, in Britain today, largely remains a pathological and defeminised process.

If Lawrence Beech is right, how do women negotiate the present system with its veneer of choice hiding increasing levels of medical control and intervention?

> *When I was pregnant with Rory I was made to feel that every thing was being done with my best interests at heart. Even when I felt unhappy about a decision, I felt I had no choice. After all they were the experts, they could see things that I knew nothing about. I just wanted a healthy baby, so I shut up and got on with it.*

> (Andrea, twenty-five-year-old woman on her first experience of maternity care)

Scrying for the future?

Twenty-first century technobaby

> *The more we technologize birth and child raising, the more the adults so raised will want to technologize their environments, the more they will extend those technologies to conception, pregnancy and birth, and child raising. And so the notion of the cyborg becomes the only hopeful way of interpreting this process, because at least, even as cyborgification mechanizes humans, it also anthropomorphizes machines.*

(Davies Floyd, 1994, p. 9)

Is the future for women to embrace technology and claim ownership over the guardians of control as tentatively suggested by Davies Floyd or is it wholesale rejection of the system? Both require a shift in the female sense of self and the ability to access power.

> *I saw my sister writhing about in agony and it was awful, it was not the picture I had in my head at all. When I was in labour with Joe I wanted everything going, no pain for me, thank you very much. Once the epidural was in, it was marvellous, I could sit and have a conversation and when it was all over, I had a bath put the slap back on and was ready to face the world.*

(Michelle, aged thirty)

Here is a woman who certainly gives the experience of knowing what she wants, or does she? Michelle knows that she does not want to be left like her sister unsupported and in pain. If that is the alternative then she does not want it. However, how many women like Michelle actually have the power to engage with the maternity systems to the extent that they are fully informed of the implications of their choices? Michelle would argue that she stated what she wanted as a consumer of services and that she controlled her birth experience. While this may be true to a certain extent, it is also possible to argue that the system left Michelle with a dichotomised view of her projected experience, where there is no real choice — only limited options. It seems that Michelle is a woman who sees what the system is really like and makes her choices on the basis of her interpretation of the system rather than on the basis of emancipatory participation and choice. Campbell and Porter (1997) would argue that the cyborg manifesto is a revamping of the traditional biomedical standpoint and as such we progress in the technocratic mechanisation process and do not address the issue of full and equal participation. If we accept the rhetoric of consumerism and choice in relation to maternity care provision are we really opening up new agendas? Or are we, like the cyborg manifesto, renaming what we already have in an attempt to make it appear new? It is possible to argue that the concept of women as consumers is an old adage. As such, the consumerist approach to childbirth could be used to give the impression of choice and control, but in effect proves to be the perfect vehicle for the current medical discourse and unequal participation of women.

> *In the dawning of the advertising era in the 1950s, the characteristic image of the woman was in the role of wife, mother or seductress. Woman as consumer was perhaps the most popular theme, the woman encouraged to believe that she needed the goods on offer in order to be fulfilled.*

(Ussher, 1991, p. 269)

In consuming without question what is currently available, are we any more empowered than our sisters in the fifties who consumed twilight sleep and the stereotypical images of femininity, until they themselves were consumed by the constraints of their own existence?

Are we not in the same place when we speak about client empowerment and participation? The adherence to the concept of empowerment is within itself an adherence to an unbalanced power relationship. For women to be empowered someone else has *de facto*, to act as the agent of empowerment. Who are those agents? Is it the medical establishment? Not according to the childbirth activists who are inundated with calls from women who have been subjected to the depersonalised and dispossessing experience of the maternity services. Is it the midwives, advocates of women and autonomous practitioners? Well, who empowered the midwives? The same issues for women as clients often afflict the most heavily gendered of all health professions, the midwives. Midwifery, the one profession that deals not just with women as the focus of care, but also women's reproduction/production.

> *When childbirth is subject to a medical definition, it is the doctors who must control childbirth not women. The implication of this — in a world where women are anything other than merely accessories to the male professional point of view — is inevitably to some extent a struggle for power.*

(Oakley, 1990, p. 9)

The relationship between midwives and the dominant medical culture around them would potentially indicate that midwifery struggles with its own identity, fighting with its own disempowerment. The disempowerment of the advocate may leave her in a position to understand and unite with the woman as client, but why have an advocate who is unable/unwilling to speak?

However, the ultimate act of consumer action is to refuse to consume. Cease to be a client. Cease to use the system.

Unassisted birth — the ultimate emancipation?

The unassisted childbirth movement appears to be a growing phenomenon in the North American continent. Women, although in small but increasing numbers, are moving away from a system which they perceive as stripping them of all dignity and innate power. This movement recognises the spirituality and power of birth and how this is corroded by contemporary western birth practices. Here the rejection of modern birth includes the rejection not just of the medical profession, but also of midwives and doulas. This women-led movement perhaps represents the ultimate in client participation and emancipation — the right to reject all other alternatives. Does this represent a possible alternative in the future for women in Britain, or are we culturally too far removed from the North American birth system to follow suit? It could be argued that we are on the same path as North America and that we will eventually adopt their birth trends, although usually this argument is made with technology and medicalisation in mind.

Perhaps unassisted birth as an alternative is nearer than we think. Few women, as yet, are fully aware of their birth rights; the system has done a good job of ensuring that they remain uninformed. The health professionals are in such conflict with each other that the women find themselves lost in the middle of a battle for power. The rates of homebirth remain relatively low across the country and few women step outside the system to use independent midwives or medical private practice. Up until fairly recently women have relied on their local professionals and networks for information and support; the media itself is limited in the portrayal of birth choices. However, the Internet provides access to anyone on almost any subject; access through the home or through public services such as the library. For the many women who could utilise that access it may be the opening to new ways of knowing, new ways of accessing professionals or lay groups who do not follow the dominant ideology.

> *It is the users of the Internet information rather than authors or professional experts who decided what and how material is accessed and used — the Internet forms the site of a new struggle over expertise in health that will transform the relationship between health professionals and their clients.*

(Hardey, 1999, p. 820)

This access to information includes not only the women who anticipate a normal birth but also those women where there are known medical problems or fetal problems. Currently, these are the women who have a harder time retaining choice and active participation in the care process as access to information is difficult and dependency upon the professionals is at a premium.

The future is more than a dichotomy of extremes in a society that continually reinvents itself; there must be a future that involves more than outright rejection or submission.

Equal participation/ownership of provision

Perhaps we need to re-look at the present and see what else is happening that may portend well for the future. The Royal College of Midwives published *Vision 2000* (RCM, 2000) to look at the potential future of the maternity services. Although the focus of the document is upon where midwifery will be in the maternity provision of the future, the ethos is that of partnership between the woman and the health professionals involved in her care.

> *It is not good enough to rely on established relationships with user groups, or women's feedback on existing patterns of provision, or on the voices of those who are articulate*

or forceful enough to make themselves heard — useful as all these are. The voices of those women whose outcomes are poorest — and who are most in need of appropriate and flexible maternity care — are rarely heard, and the maternity service must find ways to rectify that — notwithstanding the obvious problems of securing informed and confident contributions, ensuring that all sectors of the community are represented, avoiding tokenism, and breaking down professional protectionism.

(RCM, 2000, p. 7)

It can be argued that pregnancy and childbirth are public health issues and, as such, very much a part of current government agendas. Where women are actively involved in developing service provision the outcomes have been positive, such as the development of a new birthing unit at Newbury. Women are encouraged to play an active part in the management of the Edgeware Birth Centre in Middlesex (Walker, 2000). In the late 1980s, birthing facilities closed around the country, but it would appear that they are back on the agenda again. This time the difference is that women want to participate in such schemes and midwives are very much aware that without the pressure from the clients, even the best of schemes are doomed to failure in a cut throat healthcare arena where everyone competes for their share.

The thought of giving birth in that place is too much, why can't I have my baby somewhere accessible and friendly? Somewhere where you feel that you are safe.

(Diane, aged twenty-four years)

Most women currently still want to give birth in hospital as the propaganda against homebirth has been too persuasive. But, the women themselves may lead maternity provision back into the community where it can be argued to belong. It may be possible to argue that women still want the current paternalistic service where decisions are made for them by people 'who know best'. Why have experts if you do not utilise their skills? However, the removal from the decision-making process, is a removal from self-determination and responsibility. This then transcends the concept of expertise and fosters a different set of power relations, which is inherently imbalanced and unhealthy. Client participation at whatever level that individual is able, is paramount to self-determination and a crucial part of birth and the passage to parenthood.

> *It should be remembered that the success or failure of organisational structures and systems is critically dependent on whether those working within them want them to succeed or fail. While change is essential if the maternity services are to fulfil their potential, this change must be owned by those who provide and receive the care, as well as by those who plan it and pay for it.*

(RCM, 2000, p. 13)

Birthing realities

The maternity services have undergone a series of changes over the past thirty years and although some of this change can be attributed to the changing policies and politics of health care, the presence of a strong and articulate activist movement has at least stemmed part of the tide of medicalisation and most definitely ensured that the rights of women as clients is never far from the agenda.

Although the presence of articulate and well-organised groups such as AIMS and the NCT have been dismissed as middle class and removed from the reality of most women's experiences, without their presence, the provision of maternity care today would be far poorer. The reality is that the majority of women in this country will at some time in their lives, at least once, come into contact with the maternity services. The majority of those women are not ill and they are anticipating what is generally seen as a normal event in the life of a woman. This means that there is a potentially large activist base within society to change and protest — a large amount of potential voters to appease and win over. The politicising of women through the feminist movement has resulted in the politicising of childbirth, and service providers would be well advised to think beyond the confines of hospital politics and look to the broader social agenda of women as agents for social change.

Key points

✳ Childbirth and motherhood are pivotal features of many women's lives, regardless of ethnicity, class or background. The decisions to have children, not to have children, or to delay parenthood are all features of contemporary British society.

✳ Ethnicity, class and background will without doubt effect the expectations of a woman and her family group, and the nature of interaction between the pregnant woman and the service providers.

✳ Social class and ethnicity are factors that directly influence the type of care that women are likely to receive, in terms of information, choice and intervention.

✳ The growth and rhetoric of consumerism within the field of childbirth suggests some level of dissonance between providers of care, policy makers and the women receiving care provision.

✳ Consumer groups such as the NCT are actively surveying their membership and using the information gained to try and change the quality of maternity care received by women.

References

Audit Commission (1997) *First Class Service: improving maternity services in England and Wales.* Audit Commission, London

Bluff R, Holloway I (1994) 'They know best': Women's perceptions of midwifery care during labour and childbirth. *Midwifery* **10**: 157–64

Campbell R, Porter S (1997) Feminist theory and the sociology of childbirth: A response to Ellen Annandale and Judith Clark. *Sociology of Health and Illness* **19**(3): 348–58

Clinical Standards Advisory Group (1995)*Women in Normal Labour.* HMSO, London

Commission for Racial Equality (1994) *Race Relations Code of Practice in the Maternity Services.* Caxton House Press Limited, London: 9

Cooper Y (2000) *Debate on Maternity Care.* Hansard Report, 19April

Lawrence Beech B (1999/2000) Over medicated and under informed: What are the consequences for birthing women? *Aims Journal* **11**(4): 4–7

Davies-Floyd R (1994) *Inner space and outer space as cyberspace: technocratizing womb and world.* Paper presented at the annual meeting of the American Anthropological Association, December :9

Department of Health (1993) *Changing Childbirth: Report of the expert maternity group.* DoH, London

Department of Health (1991) *Patient's Charter.* DoH, London

Green JM, Kitzinger JV, Coupland VA (1990) Stereotypes of childbearing women: A look at some evidence. *Midwifery* **6**: 125–32

Hardey M (1999) Doctor in the House: The Internet as a source of lay health knowledge and the challenge to expertise. *Sociology of Health and Illness* **21**(6): 820–35

Maternity Action in Leicestershire (1996) *Changing Childbirth Users Forum.* News Letter, November: 1

McCourt C, Page L, eds (1996) *Report on the evaluation of one-one midwifery.* TVU , London

National Childbirth Trust (1990) *What women want from midwives, obstetricians, general practitioners, health visitors and anaesthetists*. NCT/Alexandra House, London: 5

National Childbirth Trust (1994) *Maternity Services Charter Out of Sight?* NCT Press Release

National Health Service Executive (1997) *The new NHS — modern, dependable*. DoH, London

Oakley A (1986) *The Captured Womb*. Blackwell, Oxford: 251

Oakley A (1990) Foreword. In: Pratten B *Power, Politics and Pregnancy*. Health Rights Limited, London

Reid M (1992) *The disappearance of homebirth. Paper delivered to the Second International Homebirth Conference*. Sydney, Australia, October: 3

Royal College of Midwives (2000) *Vision 2000*. RCM Press, London

Sheahan D (1972) The game of the name, nurse professional and nurse technician. *Nurs Outlook* **20**: 440–4

Ussher J (1991) *Women's Madness: Misogyny or Mental Illness?* Harvester Wheatsheaf, London: 269

Walker J (1999) BUMPS up and running. *Midwifery Matters* **82**: 4–6

Walker J (2000) *Presentation on the Edgeware Birth Centre. Inaugural meeting of the Birth Centre Network*. Birmingham Women's Hospital

Winterton N (2000) *Debate on Maternity Care*. Hansard Report, 19 April: 2

Zadorosnzj M (1999) Social class, social selves, and social control in childbirth. *Sociology of Health and Illness* **21**(3): 267–89

5

Empowerment and participation versus social control: local authority social work with children and families

Tony Booth

Introduction

In North America in 1874 there were laws against the ill treatment of animals but no laws to protect children. When a little girl called Mary Ellen was found neglected, beaten and cut in a New York tenement, it was argued and established in court that she was entitled to protection due to her being a member of the animal kingdom (Cloke and Davis, 1997). We've come a long way since then... or have we?

> *Why do kids in care feel shitty? No one tells them they love them. No one tells them they're good at anything. No one encourages them to be good at anything.*

(Child A, speaking from personal experience)

This book focuses on the extent to which users of healthcare services feel involved in decisions made by those services — participation; and the extent to which they feel in control of their interactions with those services — empowerment. This chapter focuses on issues of participation and empowerment in service users' experience of local authority child care social work.

Social control and vested interests

In comparison with other fields of health care, issues of participation and empowerment are of special significance in social work for at least three reasons. Firstly, when a patient is using health care to deal with a physical ailment the interaction between user and healthcare agency is a tool which facilitates the delivery of the core service, the treatment. If a patient experiences his or her interactions with a hospital consultant to be disempowering, she/he may feel this is a price worth paying to be cured. In much of social work, practice, the interaction between user and agency workers, is often in itself the core service; it is the cure.

Secondly, those persons who use social services are typically among the most disempowered people in society. The very fact of their disempowerment is often at the root of their involvement with the service. It must follow that if those persons do not feel empowered by their interactions, then their service user status is likely to be perpetuated.

Thirdly, central aspects of social work with children and families are bound up with issues of social control — on the face of it, the antithesis of empowerment. Social work can be seen as the 'sticking plaster' of the state, covering over the wounds of deprivation, poverty and oppression, helping society to be healthy or at least helping to create the illusion of a society in acceptable health. These social control functions are especially manifest in the most high profile and potentially sensitive aspects of child care social work, ie. child abuse and children in care, or to use the technical and legal terminology, child protection and 'looked after' children.

Social workers can be seen as the 'soft police', supervising and constraining individuals and groups perceived to be a threat to society. Save for those occasions when the media have a good story to tell, eg. abuse of children in care or a child killed by abusive parents, the public as a whole has relatively little knowledge of, or interest in, the activities of child care social workers. What goes on behind closed doors does not directly affect their quality of life, but they would sooner have dirty or delinquent children safely tucked away in care than roaming the streets.

The state has a vested interest in maintaining the notion that the greatest damage to children arises, on the one hand, out of poor parenting and, on the other, out of social services' failure to protect children, or to look after them properly. In reality, it is the structural inequalities and power imbalances in society which cause far greater damage. It seems that social services departments are expected to collude with this illusion. One senior manager in a Midlands local authority, charged with drafting a paper for submission to the National Society for the Prevention of Cruelty to Children (NSPCC) Commission on the Prevention of Child Abuse, wrote:

It is possible when one considers such issues as child poverty, poor housing, polluted environments, inadequate public health provision, absence of affordable child care,

> *and social and racial discrimination, to talk about*
> *structural abuse and to suggest that the damage caused by*
> *these factors far outweighs the damage caused by more*
> *individual-based notions of child abuse.*

Interestingly, this paragraph appeared in the initial draft but was deleted from the final submission!

If neither the public nor the state has any real interest in the genuine empowerment of the victims of structural inequality, what about social workers themselves? Most come into social work in part through some broad notion of wanting 'to help people'. There is not a huge gap between saying, 'I want to help people' and saying, 'I feel good if people depend upon me'. They are not inevitably the same thing, but they clearly can be. Genuine empowerment of social services' users may deprive social workers of the warm satisfaction of 'doing good'.

At the professional level, genuine empowerment threatens professional autonomy and the notion of the expert. When I sat recently with a family going through the social worker's report, I read that, '... it is clear that (the child's) challenging behaviour arises out of a degree of attachment deficit combined with the parents' dysfunctional approaches to behaviour management'. My comment to the (semi-literate) parents, 'Don't worry if you don't understand this, because neither do I', seemed to set them at ease. They participated actively in the meeting; the social worker did not say another word.

The state we're in

Participation and empowerment are concepts that social workers may come across in their training courses — although less so in recent years as training becomes progressively de-politicised — but which make little impact on real life social work at the coal face. Social work involvement in the lives of children and families has unintended and disempowering negative consequences. These consequences include pathologisation, stigmatisation, dependency creation and social control. A logical corollary is that social work professionals should take steps to avoid these negative consequences. Arguably, they should only intervene at the minimum level necessary to achieve the minimum acceptable level of change. Such thinking, known as 'minimum necessary intervention', developed in the late sixties and through the seventies from the writings of radical academics on the left such as Stan Cohen and Jock Young. These practice principals subsequently gained credence, but for different reasons, with politicians on the right. The notion of minimum necessary intervention became compatible with Thatcherite rhetoric about 'rolling back the frontiers of the state'. It also provided convenient academic justification for cutbacks in expenditure on public services.

Recent Government initiatives targeted on getting local authorities to deliver better services to children and families 'in need' have put paid to notions of minimum intervention. But the unintended consequences have not gone away. It is noticeable that rhetoric linked to participation, if not empowerment, has started to feature prominently in central and local Government statements on the future of local authority child care social work. This is not only because it provides another useful opportunity to scapegoat and demonise social workers as a distraction from the failings of Government, it is also because it is manifestly obvious that things have gone disastrously wrong.

Children in 'care'

In 1997 the Department of Health published Sir William Utting's report of a major study of the operation of the care system (Utting, 1997). In his statement to the House of Commons about the report the Secretary of State noted the following:

> *Sir William's review was necessary because of continuing revelations of widespread sexual, physical and emotional abuse of children living away from home, and in particular in children's homes over the preceding twenty years. In addition to the convictions in North Wales, there are investigations or prosecutions in progress in the North-west, the North-east, South Wales and some Home Counties.*

> *The report presents a woeful tale of failure at all levels to provide a secure and decent childhood for some of the most vulnerable children. It covers the lives of children whose home circumstances were so bad that those in authority, to use the jargon, took them into care. The*

> *report reveals that in far too many cases not enough care*
> *was taken. Elementary safeguards were not in place or not*
> *enforced. Many children were harmed rather than helped.*
> *The review reveals that these failings were not just the*
> *fault of individuals — though individuals were at fault, it*
> *reveals the failures of a whole system.*

If these words are not dramatic enough in themselves, the scale of the problem almost defies belief. *The Independent* reported on 14 September, 2000 that there were seven separate police investigations being undertaken across the UK into child abuse in care homes. These investigations involved the activities of over 1,700 suspected paedophiles. Such widespread abuse taking place unchecked over more than two decades can only have been possible if the child victims of that abuse were in a chronically disempowered position. The forces that maintained their abuse and protected the perpetrators were extremely powerful. In many of these instances the abuse was known about or suspected by a range of adults, some of whom felt unwilling or unable to speak out, or who found their concerns were not taken seriously or were inadequately investigated. Some perpetrators were protected by virtue of their powerful and respected position in society. Others were protected by employment practices ostensibly designed to protect employees from victimisation by their employer, eg. unproven allegations were expunged from the employee's records and a pattern of concerns and allegations could therefore not be established.

The abuse was even perpetuated by arguments based around the rights of the child. An organisation known as the Paedophile Information Exchange (PIE) promoted the notion that sexual contact between children and care staff should not be seen as abusive. Members of PIE, including certain prestigious child care professionals, argued that society oppressed the natural expression of sexuality by children, and that sexual contact with care staff could free them from this oppression and enhance their development.

I have focused so far on only one aspect of the failure of social services departments in relation to children 'in care', although a dramatic and tragic one. It should not be thought that for other children in care who have not been abused that the outcomes have been broadly positive. By any measure, the outcomes for 'Looked After' children have varied between poor and disastrous. Given the part that education can play in providing an escape from disadvantage, statistics on educational attainment may be seen as providing one measure of the level of empowerment of 'Looked After' children. The National Child Development study (Cheung and Heath, 1994) showed that in 1981, 43% of children in care left school with no academic qualifications. This compared with 16% of a matched sample of non-care school leavers. More recent studies have indicated that this may have been an optimistic estimate with some researchers suggesting that as few as 25% of care leavers manage to gain even one GCSE. Around 40% of children who leave care are without employment.

Child protection

Social services child protection systems and procedures exist primarily to deal with the neglect and abuse of children within their own families. Let us consider whether those systems have operated in ways that have served to challenge and promote the position of the most vulnerable and disempowered members of society. Sadly, the evidence from research is not encouraging.

A number of research studies have shown that families are typically devastated by the experience of child protection investigations and child protection case conferences. While very worrying, these findings would be a little easier to take if these processes were hitting the right target and protecting children. On the contrary, a series of research studies have concluded that many families have been inappropriately drawn into child protection systems. For example, Gibbons *et al* (1995) investigated the factors which most influenced decisions about child protection registration. They found that harm to the child had a less significant influence than did a whole range of other factors related to parental characteristics and behaviour. Prominent influences included; mental illness, domestic violence, a criminal record, drug abuse and financial problems. Thorpe (1994), a prominent social science researcher, referred to a number of similar studies conducted in three different continents over the previous ten years. He noted that child protection systems:

> ... are being used to impose standardised forms of parenting on diverse populations rather than to protect children from injury or harm.

Local authority child protection systems are highly proceduralised and time-consuming to operate. As a consequence, they eat up resources in ways which mean little is left to attend to families in need of support. Section 17 of the Children Act 1989 established a statutory duty upon local authorities to provide services to children in need. In practice, the emphasis upon child protection has drained away resources and in a context of overall budgetary restraint this has meant little capacity to meet this statutory duty. We have ended up in the paradoxical situation whereby those persons who do not want a service end up receiving one, while those who do want a service are denied help.

Ms F had found herself at one time on the receiving end of child protection enquiries, and at another time seeking help to deal with sustained emotional and behavioural difficulties with her children.

> *They didn't help me to know how I could help Matthew. He was pissing in cupboards and all sorts and they didn't help me one bit. It took them weeks to get round to letting me know they weren't going to do bugger all. I begged them for help and all I got was 'No, it's not serious enough'. Then all it took was one small problem mentioned by one official person and it was like, 'We must deal with this'. So there was a case conference and there's all these official people and it's just you and I was so scared. Even then they were more concerned about being able to wrap up their files and close the case than about helping me. I needed someone to teach me what to do, not some bossy boots telling me how to run my life, but once they decided it wasn't serious, that was it, I was on my own again.*

Empowerment: why bother?

The state of affairs described above is clearly unacceptable and in that sense 'something must be done'. But, given the powerful vested interests at work, perhaps the motivation is more to give the appearance of doing something rather than actually taking steps that genuinely change the balance of power?

Many local authorities have produced policy documents and practice guidance about consulting and involving service users in the planning and delivery of children's services. One such document lists reasons why social services need to consult and involve people.

The reasons include the following:

> ❖ It is a statutory duty of local authorities and is a key theme of recent Government legislation and guidance.
>
> ❖ It is a very powerful way to improve the quality of services and it increases people's choices and control over their lives.
>
> ❖ It makes the department more accountable for its services and encourages openness and honesty, allowing people to work together and feel ownership of the opportunities, issues and problems.
>
> ❖ It leads to the best use of public money. It helps to ensure that services are appropriate, highlights good practice that can be built on, and identifies bad practice that can be dealt with.

So far so good. How are these laudable aims to be achieved? The practice principles to be adopted include the following:

> ❖ We will recognise that service user views and carer views are potentially different.
>
> ❖ We will conduct consultation in a relevant, friendly and meaningful way that encourages participation.
>
> ❖ We will work with other departments, local agencies and groups, to ensure that good practice is shared as much as possible and avoid any duplication.
>
> ❖ We will acknowledge that consultation is not cheap and provide resources where possible to encourage involvement, including reimbursement of expenses at the appropriate times.
>
> ❖ We will recognise that consultation and involvement means users, carers and staff 'sharing power'. Training for staff, users and carers, along with provision of advocacy support and recognising the barriers to involvement, will be essential in making it work.

The document then goes on to state that, 'the Department is committed to using a variety of methods in order to facilitate consultation'. Among the methods it states should be considered are:

> ❖ Consultation days, meetings and workshops held in accessible venues at relevant times.
>
> ❖ Surveys (could be face-to-face, by telephone or by postal questionnaires, taking account of specific communication requirements).

In some ways, the above extracts are quite informative. They draw attention to some of the elements that could well form part of a participation and empowerment strategy. It will, however, come as no surprise to those readers familiar with 'local-government speak' that, in practice, all of the above has no discernible impact on the delivery of children's services in the department in question. Most child care workers in the department are either unaware of or have forgotten the existence of this document. The practice principles in particular are classic examples of the vacuous attitudinal posing that litters local authority statements of good intent. The methods for facilitating consultation remain largely unrealised. The inevitability of this no-change outcome becomes apparent once one realises that nowhere in the document is there any indication of who will take responsibility for driving this forward, no detail about resources to be made available to service these processes, and in particular no plans for any monitoring of the implementation of the commitments made.

It should be emphasised that this is not a criticism targeted at the local authority in question. A similar position will prevail in many other local authorities across the country. I am hardly the first person to draw such conclusions. Williamson and Butler (1997), authors involved in academia but also with strong connections to contemporary practice in the field, wrote:

> *We are acutely aware that while policy documents and scholarly texts may be riddled with rhetorical and appealing references to concepts such as choice, opportunity, participation, consultation, justice and empowerment, such language and aspirations are increasingly dismissed by those at the sharp end of practice as 'all gesture and no substance'. In teaching, child care, youth work and related professions, we detect a distinct climate of demoralisation, stemming from the opinion that policy development bears little relation to the grounded realities of the lives of children and young people, or to the resources required to provide them with adequate and appropriate support.*

If this claim holds water then it would appear that issuing policy documents of this nature might do more harm than good.

Let us now return to the reasons why principles of empowerment and participation are promoted, if not practised, by workers, managers, academics and politicians. There are broadly two categories of rationale. One category can be termed the consumerist approach. Proponents of the consumerist approach focus on the technical aspects of service delivery. Participation is seen as a means of enhancing the efficiency, effectiveness and economy of service delivery. The notion is that the more consumers are involved in decisions about the design and delivery of services, the more likely it is that those services will appropriately meet the needs of consumers. Any engagement of service users that goes beyond cosmetic involvement will require considerable determination, ingenuity and open mindedness from the empowering organisation. This is an approach embraced by both the left and right of the political spectrum. For the left it forms a technocratic contribution to the development of social justice. For the right, it arises from an emphasis on individualism, restraining the power of the 'Nanny State'. What it does not do is to challenge at a more fundamental level questions about who holds power and how that power is used. It merely serves to preserve the status quo in a new and more acceptable form. Hence some activists, appreciating that the powerful rarely relinquished their power willingly, will have nothing to do with such conciliatory processes, preferring to challenge from the outside through assertive or militant self-advocacy.

Human rights and the rights of the child

The major alternative to the consumerist approach is an approach based firmly on principles of social justice. Such a perspective argues that much of the work of social services only serves to reinforce the oppression of the disadvantaged and argues for empowerment from a human rights perspective.

The picture is complicated by the conflict that can exist between the interests of children and the interests of their carers. While we are accustomed to thinking about rights in relation to adults, we live in a society for which notions of children's rights are barely recognised. By virtue of their age and their vulnerability, children in our society are seen as needing the protection of their carers and the state is only expected to intervene if parents and other carers are clearly abusing their position of paternalistic responsibility.

We live in a society that believes that children cannot have rights until they are old enough and mature enough to accept responsibility. We apply different standards to adults, who are afforded rights of freedom of choice, freedom of expression, freedom from discrimination and so forth, irrespective of the degree of responsibility and maturity they are able to demonstrate. As Lansdown (1997) notes, children have in general no access to money, no right to vote, no right to express an opinion or to be taken seriously, no access to the courts, no rights (except within the framework of the Children Act which requires that the child's wishes and feelings be taken into account), to challenge decisions made on their behalf, no right to make choices about their education and no legal right to physical integrity within the family. Thus 'reasonable chastisement' remains a defence for parents using corporal punishment, while the public and media express outrage if anyone tries to interfere with the 'right' of parents to hit their children.

A number of European and Scandinavian countries have outlawed physical chastisement of children. Finland has passed a law requiring parents to consult with children in reaching any major decision that affects them, subject to the child's age and understanding. The Government of our allegedly 'advanced' western democracy has been heavily criticised for its failure to put into practice the obligations incumbent upon it through its ratification of the United Nations' Convention on the Rights of the Child (Children's Rights Development Unit [CRDU], 1994).

The levels of responsibility accepted by children in many developing countries shows us that our extension of childhood into the teenage years is not a law of nature but is socially constructed. In the case of adults we accept that the exercise of rights by one individual may interfere with the rights of another. We try to negotiate these conflicts but can turn to the law and the courts where negotiation fails. By contrast, the idea that children should have rights is seen as potentially threatening to many people. The potential for conflict between the rights of children and the rights of adults is not something to be negotiated over or for the law to interfere in. The UN Convention on the Rights of the Child, Article 5, sees parents as having the responsibility to provide appropriate guidance and direction to the child, such that the child may exercise his or her rights in a manner consistent with their capacity to understand and make judgements about the issue at hand. Article 12 states that every child who is capable of forming their own view must have the right to express those views freely in all matters affecting the child.

In the UK, it is the courts rather than the Government that have, on the whole, promoted such notions. The most notable example is that of the judgement handed down in the Gillick case (*Gillick* v. *West Norfolk and Wisbech Area Health Authority* [1985]). In this instance, Lord Scarman ruled that the 'competent child has the right to consent to medical treatment irrespective of the parent's wishes'. This was a landmark judgement. This notion, that the rights of parents to make decisions on behalf of their children terminate if and when the child achieves a sufficient understanding and intelligence to enable him or her to fully understand what is proposed, has become known as 'the Gillick principle'. The principle has come to be applied to a range of other matters outside questions of consent to treatment. The principle itself has been weakened by subsequent judgements in the Court of Appeal. Another Court found that when a child (in this instance, a sixteen-year-old anorexic) refuses consent to treatment, then a parent's consent is sufficient to allow medical intervention.

For children's rights to mean anything we need to live in a society in which the fact of children being able to influence decisions about their lives is not seen as a 'charitable gift on the part of sympathetic adults' (Lansdown, *op cit*); a society in which the onus is on adults to justify intervention rather than on the child to fight the case for control over decisions about them. Such a society would see the infringement of children's rights to be as unacceptable as it now sees the infringement of the rights of women or of black people. Legally, such a society would provide properly recognised procedures for ensuring the implementation of those rights, with clear means of redress that can be pursued if rights are breached.

Ways forward

Access to information

One cannot be in the position of an informed decision-maker without access to information. The information which professionals possess tilts the balance of power in their favour. In this respect children are doubly disadvantaged, rarely having the kind of access to information that adults in general have, let alone professionals. If children are to have a genuine opportunity to participate in decisions about their lives they need information appropriate to their age and understanding, along with the opportunity and time to explore options, weigh up arguments and form a view. They also need to be clear about how the decision-making processes work and by what means their views will be taken into consideration. Service users frequently find that they are involved in meetings when they do not have any real knowledge of the process or understanding of the purpose and potential outcomes.

> *It (the case conference) was worse than going to court. You've seen courts on the telly, you sort of know what to expect. At least in court you know what it's for and you know what they can do and what they can't. You can't prepare for a case conference. You've no idea what you might get asked about. What's a case conference for anyway? Is it to take your kids away? That's all you think it's for.*

(Mrs S)

The notion that attendance at a case conference can feel more disempowering than being called to account in a court of law is frankly shocking. Clearly, service users need to know more about how meetings will be run and how their voice will be heard. They need to know what sort of questions they may be asked. They need to hear full and frank information about the evidence professionals are using to inform their views and how they interpret that evidence. They need to know what sort of things the meeting will decide upon, what is the range of potential factors that would influence those decisions. They need to know the range and nature of resources and services available.

At the time of writing, local authorities are gearing up to meet the demands of a major new initiative being driven by the Department of Health, *The Framework for the Assessment of Children in Need and their Families* (DoH, 2000). This is a prescription for future practice across the country and is designed to improve and to standardise approaches to the assessment of children in need and their families. The intention is to, 'ensure a timely response and the effective provision of services'. While these aims may be laudable there is no reason to assume that the framework will have an empowering impact when put into practice. The prescription is mainly about what information is to be collected rather than about how it is collected and how it is used.

Only those practitioners who consciously prioritise the empowerment of service users will have a chance of using the framework in an empowering way. A local authority family aide was undertaking a parenting assessment with a family known to have a history of hostility towards and poor compliance with social services. She started work by giving the parents a detailed written list of the aspects of parenting she would be noting, along with practical examples to make this list come alive. As she went through the explanation of her work the parents visibly relaxed and the father commented, 'It's just common sense really'. Levels of co-operation were good and the parents were able to use the information provided to assess critically and improve their own parenting.

Influence over the context of decision making

The case conference was in a big official room in social services with a conference table and everything. It would be better if it was like in a living room with easy chairs and coffee served. They asked me if I wanted to say anything but I was too scared and then the chance was gone. It should be more like a conversation. That doesn't mean you don't take it seriously. You can have a conversation about serious things.

(Mrs S)

Service users need to have a say about where meetings are held and how meetings are to be run. Likewise, service users are not given any say over who attends meetings.

What were the police doing there? It had nothing to do with them. And then there was the head-teacher. What about the class teacher? He knows my daughter the best.

(Mrs S)

Venues need to be physically and psychologically accessible. Help may be needed with the costs of child care to enable attendance at meetings which take place at a time which matches the parents' commitments. Time and again I have seen afternoon case conferences wrong-footed by parents needing to leave to collect their children from school.

All of the above seems a far cry from the current situation in which even the presence of parents at meetings is still a contentious issue. It is only in the last decade that parental attendance throughout the course of a conference has become common place, and it is still not universal. Parental attendance at the inter-agency core group meetings which review and modify the child protection plan between conferences is the exception rather than the norm. Many child care professionals are resistant to such a notion. As for children in care, no one asks the child, 'How do you want these decisions to be made? Do you want to have a meeting? If so, where do you want it to be, who do you want to be there, who do you want to run it?'

Control over what work is done and how

When it comes to deciding what and how to work with service users, contemporary practice is dominated by a 'professionals know best' mentality. Although written agreements between workers and service users are becoming more common, whether they are used or not is generally the decision of practitioners who also determine most or all of the content (Katz, 1997). The position is made worse by the fact that some theoretical models informing social work practice actually mitigate against user participation in decision making (eg. psychodynamic theory and systems theory).

Contrast this with an approach that would be the ultimate in user empowerment — a system in which the users employ the workers. Imagine a position in which child care professionals seek to reach an understanding with parents about what needs to change and the parents are then given a certain amount of purchasing power to access those services and workers that they feel are most likely to assist them in achieving their aims.

Short of such a radical re-think in the delivery of child care social services, with the right commitment from agencies, ways can be found to give service users more control.

> *Fun and Families (a voluntary agency), were much better than social services. They said right from the beginning that I'd got eight sessions but they could be when I wanted them. I could wait a month or I could ring up and say I needed one sooner.*

(Ms F)

Effective communication with service users

It is self-evident that effective communication is necessary in order to solicit the views of service users. In respect of adults, I consider below some of the steps which can increase the opportunity for their voice to be heard. There are additional issues for children.

Most of us like to think that we are experts on children, 'after all, I was one myself once'. But this is part of the problem. Because we believe that we are experts we tend not to believe that we can learn much of value by actually listening to what children have to say. Such listening needs to take account of the fact that the issues most pertinent to the child may be very different from those which concern the professionals. Adults need to be prepared to pay attention to the child's agenda, even when it seems to them relatively trivial. Only when children are consulted over the little decisions as part of day-to-day experience, will they feel sufficiently empowered to participate in the big decisions.

The professional's personal style is especially important when communicating with children, as is vividly demonstrated by the research of Williamson and Butler (1997). One of their findings that will come as no surprise to anyone who genuinely understands children is that, 'children and young people make quick judgements as to whether an individual adult is "all right", or is a "dickhead" '. They found that children's assessment of adults, and their assessment of whether an adult is worth proper communication with, were at least in the initial stages of contact based on 'maverick qualities of which humour was a central part. Being a "good laugh" was a critical attribute. What young people sought from adults was some serious listening inside a funny shell'.

Some adults have the knack of connecting with children very quickly. Others present a persona that children feel is utterly alien. Williamson and Butler (*op cit*) note that textbooks rarely make any reference to the qualities that really help to connect with children. They draw a contrast between the communication style proposed by the American National Institute of Justice, 'I wonder whether it feels scary to talk to a stranger about stuff that is so hard to talk about?' — and the kind of approach they found worked the best — 'Come on, I bet you're the first to moan that no-one ever listens to you. Well I'm right here ready to listen to anything you have to say'. They found that humour and self-effacement were useful personal attributes to take into an interview.

Factors that are more likely to be referred to by social work texts are those of gender and ethnicity. In the research quoted above, contingency arrangements were established to ensure that any child who so wished could be interviewed by a researcher of the same gender or ethnicity. In the event, the contingency arrangements were not required. White males conducted all interviews. The young people concerned were strikingly firm and unanimous that the issue for them was whether or not the researcher seemed to understand where they were coming from, and they were determined they would make up their own mind about this. This is not to throw the baby out with the bath water. It is crucially important that child care workers take care to establish the preferred language of communication for both adults and children. This includes access to interpreters, use of sign language, use of large print media, etc. Effective communication means establishing quickly what will work best with any one individual rather than following formulae from textbooks or policy documents. Educationalists are familiar with the notion that different people learn best through different approaches; some work best with spoken language, some with written language and some through non-linguistic channels, including pictures and signs, touch, or experiential learning. The primary limiting factor is the ingenuity and determination of the worker concerned.

One social worker's case involved a child with severe learning difficulties, no speech and very little sign language. The child had been provided with a special corset in order to sit upright and to slow down degeneration of her congenitally malformed spine. Parents chose not to use the corset at home, claiming the child was distressed by its use. The social worker was determined to take her own steps to establish the wishes and feelings of the child and became the only person outside the family to observe the child in several different settings, with and without the corset. She found that wearing the corset the child was alert and engaged with her surroundings, gurgling and smiling. Without it she was disengaged and isolated. The determination of the social worker gave the child a voice in the decision-making process, freeing the child from unnecessary physical and mental distress.

Service user feedback

Much of what is said above about communication also applies to soliciting user feedback about service provision. There are a few extra points worth making. Firstly, the will to solicit feedback is crucial. While the Government regularly promotes the notion that local authorities design services partly on the basis of user feedback, it does not provide a very good model in its own practice. Take, for example, the Government's preparation of its first report to the United Nations Committee on the Rights of the Child. Cloke (1997) reports that in producing the report the Government did not consult with either children and young people or with non-governmental organisations. He contrasts this with the performance of the Children's Rights Development Unit which simultaneously produced its own report but which undertook an extensive consultation exercise involving children and young people and statutory and voluntary organisations.

A second point is that child care workers, frequently with the support of their Trade Unions, are willing to participate in feedback exercises but only so long as they are designed in ways which do not identify individual workers. In an era where employers are increasingly embracing performance assessment, it seems extraordinary that employers and employees alike are colluding in the avoidance of feedback on an issue which is of such critical importance to service users — how they are treated by individual professionals.

Thirdly, in order for user feedback to make a difference, the feedback needs to be received at all levels of the organisation and in ways which are likely to have the greatest impact. Charts and statistics may be most appropriate in terms of influencing senior managers concerned with wider issues of policy and resource planning. For workers at the 'coal-face', individual testaments delivered to a team meeting, with ex or current service users talking about their experiences, may have a far greater impact.

Self-esteem, mutual support and self-advocacy

The people most needing social service provisions are often among the most vulnerable members of society. They are often the least able to put feelings into words, least accustomed to having their views respected, and most easily overawed or intimidated by figures of authority and by bureaucratic agencies. Poor self-esteem results in individuals who are unlikely to take power readily and likely to have their self-esteem further damaged by contact with social services. This is particularly true of those for whom poor self-esteem is linked to lack of self-identity, as can more frequently be the case with service users from ethnic minorities and with children in care who have lost contact with their family of origin.

The experience of being listened to and taken seriously can in itself enhance self-esteem. Some individuals may benefit from work specifically targeted on raising self-esteem in order to take more control over their lives. Considerably greater empowerment can often be experienced by coming together in groups along with others who have had similar experiences or are facing similar difficulties. Users can experience a sense of strength in numbers, feeling that they are not alone, sharing experiences, feelings and ideas, providing mutual support and taking the opportunity to form a collective view of service provision. Social services are in a position to encourage the development of such groups, enabling people to get in touch with other persons in similar circumstances, making available venues, helping with transport and so forth. There needs to be an understanding that even when a group starts with a focus on mutual support, as participants gain in confidence the group may shift its focus towards self-help and self-advocacy. If such groups end up mounting a powerful challenge to the status quo of service provision, the true test of the organisation arises. Does it respond positively to the challenge or does it accuse its accusers of biting the hand that feeds them?

External advocacy

In the conference I was all alone. In court you've got a solicitor to back you up and give you advice.

(Mrs S)

If a service user turns up to a case conference with a solicitor they are generally seen as choosing an adversarial approach. The exception to this is when the service user is known to be prone to aggression, in which case the presence of a solicitor is welcomed as a means of keeping the service user calm. There can be few more telling examples of the tendency of the agency to think in ways that place greater importance on keeping control than on effective communication with service users.

When it comes to care proceedings, in recognition of the importance of ensuring that the child's interests and wishes are represented, courts appoint a *Guardian Ad Litem* whose job it is to specifically represent the interests of the child. Contrast this with a case conference that was considering a circumstance in which a child with significant learning difficulties and challenging behaviour had received a series of physical injuries. The parents acknowledged that they were probably responsible for the injuries but argued that they were caused in the process of self-defence and necessary restraint of their child. Despite the fact that the residential school where the child lived during the week had never 'needed' to cause any physical injury to the child, conference members concluded no registration or other protective action was appropriate — not even training for the parents in appropriate restraint. Conference members felt great sympathy for the parents in having to care for this burdensome child and were disinclined to do anything that might put them under greater 'pressure'. The no-action decision was subsequently reconsidered and modified but only because of the presence at the conference of a welfare professional who also happened to be the parent of a disabled child. With the support of her manager she dissented from the conference decision and advocated from the child's perspective.

A recently published research overview (Sinclair and Franklin, 2000) notes that the Department of Health guidance encourages social services to enable children in care to bring supporters or independent advocates to their reviews. Despite this encouragement, they reported that 'it rarely happens'. Invitations to children to attend child protection case conferences are not common practice, yet where local authorities do actively encourage attendance, children have responded positively. In one study, 80% of children, mostly aged twelve or over, attended (Sinclair and Franklin, *op cit*).

There are particular circumstances in which life-changing decisions are likely to be made on behalf of those least able to represent their own views. Child protection case conferences and 'Looked After' children reviews are two examples. We need to live in a society in which lack of advocacy in such situations is as unusual as going into a house purchase or divorce without a solicitor.

Trust and confidentiality

> *The Fun and Families worker was all right. She wasn't judgmental. Social services just snooped around and then closed the file. Then every time you've got a problem and you ring up, you speak to someone different. You never get to know or trust someone and they haven't got time to read the case notes.*
>
> (Ms F)

Without the opportunity to build trusting relationships with child care professionals it is difficult to see how relationships between service users and social services can be anything but problematic. This is a particular problem for 'Looked After' children, who frequently experience changes of social worker and, for many of whom, there is little stability in placements either. It is difficult to parent a child properly if there is no continuity of carer. One of the current Government objectives in its 'Quality Protects' programme is to, 'Reduce to no more than 16% in all authorities by 2001, the number of children "Looked After" who have three or more placements in one year' (DoH, 1999). The fact that this is an ambitious target says much about the current position of many children in care in terms of establishing relationships of trust with their carers.

Issues of confidentiality are linked to issues of trust. Social services set a high priority on confidentiality. But what the agency means by confidentiality may be at variance with the service user's notion.

> *They didn't trust us (ie. service user and her husband) in saying, 'We've dealt with it, we've talked with him (their son) and sorted it out'. They insisted on talking to him themselves. We didn't want them to but in the end we went along with it 'cos they (ie. social services) were threatening to ring up the headmaster of the school. I didn't want him labelled a pervert at school.*

(Mrs S)

Most service users will accept the notion that other persons and agencies will at times need to have information passed to them from social services. However, they will generally expect that this is done on a 'need to know' basis. This is not the same as sharing information on the 'might need to know' basis which typifies current practice. Jack (1997) refers to research showing that children and young people are very disinclined to share information with teachers, social workers, youth workers, etc. because they could not trust them not to 'spread it around'. Child care social workers generally take it for granted that confidentiality is not an issue. This is not how service users see it. The challenge is to provide a service that matches users' notions of confidentiality.

Procedures to serve the people, not people to serve the procedures

In an attempt to maintain minimum standards of practice, local authority social work is becoming increasingly procedurally driven. In a climate of fear, where politicians and the tabloid press delight in the opportunities for 'social worker bashing', it is not surprising that managers have sought to proceduralise out the potential for error. This is an approach doomed to failure, as decades of enquiries into child deaths have shown. Most of the issues I have identified above cannot be tackled via procedures. There are no substitutes for personal commitment and sound judgement.

Regrettably, there are times when procedures not only fail to make things better but end up making things worse. This is because they are used inflexibly, with individuals not being allowed to use their own judgement and discretion where procedures seem unhelpful. Chris Wilson (1997) refers to a boy who had six foster homes in two years but then settled in a foster home where at last he was happy. Then one day 'Mum' (the foster carer) smacked him when he stole money from her purse. The next day he was removed, irrespective of the fact that he desperately wanted to stay and the foster carer was happy to continue caring for him. The boy found himself in a new placement where he was most unhappy and faced a further history of serial placement breakdown. A procedure designed to protect children from abusive carers, inflexibly applied, served to cause more harm than the harm it was trying to prevent.

Some procedures are perpetuated despite evidence of their inappropriateness. For several years now there have been national practice standards for the videoing of children who are being interviewed about being abused. The intention behind these procedures was to reduce the need for children to be required to give evidence-in-chief under cross-examination during criminal trials of alleged abuse perpetrators. Such experiences had distressed and damaged children and many perpetrators had escaped justice thanks to the ability of the defence to break down child witnesses in court. The laudable intentions of the procedures have, in practice, been threatened by a variety of (mainly legal) factors. By 1993, approximately 15,000 video interviews had been conducted; only forty-four had been accepted as evidence in court (Cohen, 1993). Yet the procedures remained in place, with all the potential for stress and distress inherent in children talking about highly personal and traumatic experiences before two strangers and a video camera.

A fundamental change of attitude is needed in respect of procedures. They need to be a tool that facilitates good practice, not a straight jacket that constrains the capacity for professional judgement. Service users' views should not end up as just one element of procedural consideration but instead should, where possible, form the cornerstone for action by social services.

Avenues for complaint and redress

It seems appropriate to conclude on the opportunity for service users to have action taken when they are ill served by social services. The right to be heard and the other rights and recommendations referred to in this chapter are meaningless without the opportunity to challenge circumstances, where those rights are breached.

The Children Act 1989 established complaints procedures as a statutory requirement. Prior to implementation of the Act, some people predicted that social services departments would be flooded by frivolous and malicious complaints. Lansdown (1997) refers to research published in 1992 by 'Voice for the Child in Care' which indicated that, 'over 80% of complaints by children have been upheld and there was, in those cases, serious justification for the complaint'. Despite this finding a recent research overview (Sinclair and Franklin, 2000) reports upon one study which indicated that 38% of children in care are unaware of the complaints procedures. Only a minority of complaints was dealt with within the required twenty-eight days (various studies suggest between 8% and 27%) and these delays were in themselves a major source of dissatisfaction for service users. We need to see a robust, accessible, well-publicised, fast moving, non-bureaucratic, user and advocate friendly, complaint and redress service.

At least complaints services do exist and are being used. Many of the other ways forward that I have identified above require major shifts in power relationships. It seems that there is much to be done. Optimism for the future would be, I fear, a triumph of hope over experience.

Tony Booth

Key points

⌘ The price of disempowerment is traditionally the cost we pay for care in statutory services.

⌘ People who use social services are typically disempowered and their utilisation of these services is often a symptom of an inability to advocate for themselves.

⌘ The antithesis of empowerment is social control.

⌘ The process of child protection in itself may be destructive and often deleterious to both the family and the child.

⌘ 'The professionals know best' mentality perpetuated by the professionals themselves should be questioned in both training and fieldwork.

⌘ Children have rights before they are mature enough to take responsibility.

References

Cheung S, Heath A (1994) Aftercare — the education and occupation of adults who have been in care. *Oxford Review of Education* **20**: 361–74

Children's Rights Development Unit (1994) *UK Agenda for Children*. CRDU, London

Cloke C (1997) Forging the circle: the relationship between children, policy, research and practice in children's rights. In: Cloke C, Davies M, eds. *Participation and Empowerment in Child Protection*. Wiley, Chichester: 263–85

Cloke C, Davies M (1997) *Participation and Empowerment in Child Protection*. Wiley, Chichester

Cohen P (1993) In the frame. Children's evidence. *Community Care*, 28 October: 9

Department of Health (1999) *The Government's Objectives for Children's Social Services*. DoH, London

Department of Health (2000) *Framework for the Assessment of Children in Need and Their Families*. DoH, London

Gibbons J, Conroy S, Bell C (1995) *Operating the Child Protection System: A study of child protection practices in english local authorities*. DoH, London

Jack G (1997) Discourses of child protection and child welfare. *Br J Social Work* 27: 659–78

Katz I (1997) Approaches to empowerment and participation in child protection. In Cloke C, Davies M, eds *Participation and Empowerment in Child Protection*. Wiley, Chichester: 154–69

Lansdown G (1997) Children's rights to participation and protection: A Critique. In: Cloke C, Davies M, eds *Participation and Empowerment in Child Protection*. Wiley, Chichester: 19–38

Sinclair R, Franklin A (2000) *Young people's participation: quality protects research briefing*. Darlington Hall Trust, Darlington

Thorpe D (1994) *Evaluating Child Protection*. OU Press, Oxford

United Nations (1992) *United Nations Convention on the Rights of the Child*. Treaty Series, 44. HMSO, London

Utting W (1997) *People Like Us; Report of the review of safeguards for children living away from home*. HMSO, London

Williamson H, Butler I (1997) No one ever listens to us: Interviewing children and young people. In: Cloke C, Davies M, eds *Participation and Empowerment in Child Protection*. Wiley, Chichester: 61–79

Wilson C (1997) Issues for children and young people in local authority accommodation. In: Cloke C, Davies M, eds *Participation and Empowerment in Child Protection*. Wiley, Chichester:140–53

6

The lesbian, gay man's and transgendered experience as users of healthcare services

Jane Godfrey

The last twenty years have seen many changes in the organisation and delivery of health care. One of the central movements has been away from services planned by medical 'experts' for passive patients to the recognition that users need to be represented and heard in the process of meeting the healthcare needs of local populations and individuals. Patient participation is at least theoretically supported by such governmental papers as *The Patient's Charter* (DoH, 1991), *Working in Partnership* (DoH, 1994) and *The new NHS — modern, dependable* (DoH, 1997). This represents an enormous challenge to service providers, but there is evidence that users' involvement in heath care is evolving (Ranade, 1997; Cahill, 1998; Fraher and Limpinnian, 1999; Hickey and Kipping, 1998).

Such a fundamental change in provision is likely to be gradual and one of the areas that currently needs to be developed relates to the health care of the lesbian, gay or transgendered individual. For the purposes of this chapter, the term lesbians identifies women whose primary relationships are with women. Gay men identifies men whose primary relationships are with men. Transgendered persons include transvestites, transexuals living in identified roles and taking hormones, pre- and post-operative transexuals, and transexuals who do not want genital reconstruction.

There is a dearth of literature exploring the healthcare needs of these identified groups (Nelson, 1994; Gray *et al*, 1996, James and Platzer, 1999; Nemoto *et al*, 1999; Robertson, 1997) and much of the research is American. While the context of health care in Northern America is different from that of the United Kingdom, there are similarities in the experiences of lesbians, gay men or transgendered persons either side of the Atlantic.

The healthcare system in The United Kingdom is underpinned by the assumption that to be heterosexual is the normal, proper and fixed sexual identity. This is bolstered by social structures embedded within the establishment which uphold the heterosexual relationship as superior and correct (Godfrey, 1999). Hence, health care can be seen to be rooted in heterosexism, where heterosexism is described as the institutionalisation of the superiority of heterosexuality. Hetero-sexist power then facilitates the construct of lesbian, gay and transgendered sexualities as deviant (Stevens, 1992; Gray, 1996; Jones, 1988). Sexual identity has political, social and personal implications (Weeks, 1991), emotional, social and erotic connections (Lynch, 1993) and for lesbian, gay men or transgendered people, it also has negative meanings depending upon personal prejudices and convictions of self and others. It is clear that sexuality is an essential part of the whole person, with links to self-concept and self-esteem and that it is mediated through such structures as class, race and ethnicity.

Clearly, not every lesbian, gay man or transgendered person is identical but their sexual identities are seen as 'other' or 'deviant' in a dualistic system. Jeffrey Weeks in his book, *Sexuality* (1986), explores the historical and sociological construction of sexual identities and Raymond (1980) argues that the transgendered individual 'offers a unique perspective on sex role stereotyping in a patriarchal society'. Perhaps the most useful way of describing these 'other' positions is to use the term 'outsider' (Lorde, 1980) or 'outsider within' (Collins, 1991). Collins uses the term to describe the particular perspective that resulted from black women being exploited as domestic workers within white 'families'. 'As outsiders within, black women have a distinct view of the contradictions between the dominant group's actions and ideologies' (Collins, 1991, p. 11). If we take the liberty of applying the concept of 'outsider within' to position of lesbian, gay men or transgendered people in the context of healthcare provision, we can see that this can provide a different perspective on healthcare needs.

Within this chapter, I shall identify ways in which the 'outsider within' perspective can help generate ideas and actions that promote participation and empowerment in the healthcare process for lesbians, gay men and transgendered people and highlight factors that may hinder or facilitate this.

Contextualising the experiences of lesbian, gay men and transgendered persons within healthcare provision

Foucault (1987) argues that social reality is constituted through knowledge. However, reviewing healthcare literature reveals a distinct lack of evidence of knowledge pertaining to factors that affect the health status of lesbian, gay men and transgendered people in the United Kingdom. It would seem, that there is little acknowledged social reality for these individuals and groups within the British system of healthcare provision. This idea is further supported by the suggestion from Soper (1993) that, 'the fate of oppressed groups is not simply decided at the level of competing discourses' where discourse is 'an amalgam of material practices and forms of knowledge linked together in a non-contingent relation' (p. 34). Such groups will also be affected by the current economic and political climate. The current focus, for example, on the importance of the family highlights lesbians, gay men and transgendered people as deviant and unnatural. The debate around Section 28 of the local Government Act (1988) also shows resistance to lesbian, gay and transgendered sexual identities as normal or acceptable, in that marriage is seen as the 'ideal' and other relationships are not considered to reach this gold standard (Diva, 2000).

Once it becomes obvious that what is considered to be appropriate knowledge is only relevant for a particular section of the population, it is possible to argue for the production of other and new knowledge and for the incorporation of previously marginalised knowledge to expand social reality. Producing knowledge relating to lesbian, gay men and transgendered persons' experiences as they interface with healthcare services, not only extends social reality for these groups, but also may develop increased understanding of hitherto hidden processes that lie in heterosexism and sex role stereotyping as they affect heterosexuals. This is especially true in considering the origins of the caring professions, services originally developed to serve the interests of white, middle class men (Illich, 1976; Hugman, 1991) who were also heterosexual. Within these structures, subjugated knowledge remains excluded because of its potential to disrupt the path to absolute truth (Bailey, 1993). While knowledge of these identified groups remains subjugated, empowerment and participation will be negligible.

Alternatively, to take Foucault's idea of power as force relations (1978), the very essence of inequality engenders multiple states of power and with these states of power come multiple sites of possible resistance. Knowledge is inextricably linked to power and local centres of power develop around knowledge. While there may be, from a Foucauldian perspective, little social reality for lesbians, gay men and transgendered persons receiving or demanding health care, there is the potential to create knowledge to produce a social reality. The unspeakable becomes not just speakable but spoken:

> *... the subjugated peoples themselves have to build and create discourses and practices which are not yet there.*

> (Cain, 1993, p. 87)

We can see such discourses beginning to be generated by groups such as Stonewall, an organisation campaigning for equal citizenship rights for gay men and lesbians and GLAMS, a self-help group for gay men and lesbians affected by multiple sclerosis (Bird, 1999). Work by authors such as Raymond (1980), Rickford (1995), Robertson (1997), Godfrey (1999) and James and Platzer (1999) provide some examples of how social reality for 'outsiders within' may be promulgated. Whittle (1998) explains how the Internet is creating an 'actual' reality for transgendered persons through the development of virtual networking. Such knowledge is important in exploring the contexts in which lesbian, gay and transgendered persons live and experience the world. This process needs to be further developed, with support from funding organisations, in order that we may gain a clearer picture of the heathcare needs of these individuals, enabling empowerment and participation of individuals and groups as they access health care. James and Platzer (1999) sadly write about difficulties in gaining financial support for research identifying healthcare experiences of lesbian and gay men — a clear indication that such work is not necessarily 'valued knowledge' within a heterosexist society. Producing knowledge will not be an easy task and may well highlight continuing negative attitudes to lesbians, gay men and transgendered people as 'outsiders'. It may also prove to be politically destabilising as the dualist nature of gender is challenged.

Health in a stigmatising society

The general healthcare needs of lesbians, gay men and transgendered people are no different from those of heterosexuals. However, specific needs may develop because of the level of stigmatisation and prejudice experienced. This can lead to a sense of being devalued, reduced self-esteem and incorporation of prejudice into self-beliefs, leading to internalised homophobia. This is where the individual may experience shame, guilt and self-hatred about their sexuality, reinforced by 'voyeurism, misrepresentation and negative stereo-typing' (James and Platzer, 1999, p. 75) within society. An example of how internalised homophobia is reinforced within a heterosexist society can be seen in Mahoney's work (1999) at a private clinic offering help and advice to lesbians and gay men who wish to have children. The clinic's aim was to reduce risks around conception using artificial insemination. For one Sunday tabloid newspaper, *The Mail On Sunday*, this prompted the headline 'Scandal of single gay's baby factory' and the clinic was accused of operating '... against the spirit of the law and the regulatory framework by the President of the Conservative Family Campaign' (cited in Mahoney, 1999, p. 13). At this point in time, the clinic had only offered advice to a handful of individuals, no treatment had been given. The hidden message is that lesbian and gay men should not have access to this particular healthcare practice.

In the arena of fostering and adoption, the Children's Society has recently changed its policy of accepting lesbian and gay men as potential parents. (The policy makes no mention of transgendered persons.) This has not been without criticism and the Society argued that they should not exclude a group of people. This may appear to be a very positive step, but Valios (1999) suggests that lesbian and gay men have to overcome both unwarranted sexual connotations if they engage in the fostering/adoption process, and fears that a child brought up by same sex parents will become lesbian or gay. A more positive position by the Children's Society may have been to high-light the strong qualities that many lesbian and gay men could bring to the parenting situation as people.

For the transgendered individual, there is never the opportunity to change their sex at birth as recorded on their birth certificate. They may 'pass' as a man or as a woman in society having undergone medical intervention but their gender identity can never be legally sanctioned. Hence, sex role stereotyping may reinforce internalised homophobia and self-hatred at many levels, from legal to attitudinal. Transgendered persons may have difficulty in finding their place in society's groupings as they may also be rejected by lesbian and gay men's groups and by a heterosexual society. Raymond (1980) argues that the first 'cause' of transgendering is the gender-defined society in which we live, and the fear of being discovered as neither 'properly' male nor female pushes the individual into further surgery. She describes this as a 'fetishised logic' (p. 127) which creates deviance because healthcare providers see the problem as changing someone's appearance to fit the stereotype, rather than problematising the sex role stereotypes in which we live. She writes of the politics of the symptoms, where treatment focuses on the symptoms of the individual rather than the society. Whittle (1998) argues that 'passing' creates an inauthentic experience for the transgendered person, as the individual is often conforming to a dualistic gender stereotype and is denied the choice of being oneself.

Clearly, external values and judgements can have a profound effect on the psyche and behaviour of lesbian, gay men and transgendered individuals. Internalised homophobia and living with prejudice may result in a variety of specific healthcare needs, some of which have been documented in healthcare literature. More studies have been conducted in North America than in the United Kingdom, but all help to create a body of knowledge from the 'outsider within' perspective of lesbians, gay men and transgendered persons.

Robertson's (1997) study of twenty respondents identifies various categories that may impact on the healthcare needs of gay men. Coming to terms with being gay was highlighted. There is a poignancy in trying to come to terms with your own identity when this is perceived as deviant within society and you are exposed to negative images that relate to your own identity. Birmingham City Council refused to register a residential unit for lesbian and gay teens, and the home was subject to local protests which included the smashing of windows (Rickford, 1995). For any of the teenagers trying to come to terms with being lesbian or gay, this was an extremely negative and potentially damaging event. Coming to terms with being a lesbian or gay man may involve 'passing' as heterosexual for fear of alienation, rejection and being different (Nelson, 1997). 'Passing' will often happen in a family setting where the lesbian, gay man or transgendered person may fear eviction from the family home and may become the victim of family abuse (Nelson, 1997; Shelby, 1999). 'Passing' is itself demanding and requires continuing deception (Shelby, 1999) and self-monitoring and is described by Whittle (1998) as a 'virtual' identity because it demands pretence, 'The real world has medically, socially and legally failed to afford a place in which one can authenticate oneself as trans' (p. 392). We see that coming to terms with one's sexuality can be very difficult and may create a feeling of 'exteriority', of being outside of the dominant system, a process of potential self-devaluation and depersonalisation (Hall, 1999, p. 100).

The respondents in Robertson's study (1997) also identified the development of self-worth as impacting on health. Lynch (1993) suggests that self-worth and acceptance for many lesbians involves disclosure of sexual orientation, and Loulan (1984) argues that disclosure can help to overcome internalised homophobia. For many lesbians, gay men and transgendered persons, disclosure can have a major impact on health. Robertson (1997) describes how the fear of disclosure or discovery results in gay men continually 'monitoring behaviour' and being 'hypervigilant' (p. 34). Stevens and Hall (1988) illustrate the irony involved in disclosure:

> *While self-disclosure is generally considered to be necessary in the formation of authentic interpersonal relationships (Jourard, 1971), the potential negative consequences in the behaviour of others often act as effective deterrents to self-disclosure by lesbian women.*

> (Stevens and Hall, 1988, p. 70)

Coming to terms with being a lesbian, gay man or transgendered person is fraught with difficulties within oneself and those imposed externally. The process involves developing a sense of worth and self-acceptance, but also includes self-monitoring for self-preservation. These complex processes can cause fatigue, trauma and ill health (Hall, 1999) as they access care, or as they work within the healthcare setting. Many of these experiences are disempowering and silencing. To begin to empower lesbians, gay men and trans-gendered persons, we need to break the silence and give voice to those who have been, and are still being, silenced.

Lesbians, gay men and transgendered persons engaging in health care

Reported experiences

There is no singular identity for lesbians, gay men or transgendered persons. Differences exist between individuals, as they do between heterosexual, bisexual and celibate persons, but the available literature suggests that there are many shared experiences, particularly between lesbians and gay men. As lesbians, gay men and transgendered persons access health care, often the first barrier to active involve-ment is found in assessment procedures. These commonly assume heterosexuality and static gender identity. Questions regarding marital/family status are prime examples. A lesbian or gay man in an established relationship may immediately feel that their relationship is devalued. They may either feel forced to 'come out' or to lie (Nelson, 1997; Robertson, 1997) as healthcare practitioners rarely ask about an individual's sexual orientation (Shelby, 1999). Fears around disclosure involve prejudice and hostility, including the risk of moralising from staff, of receiving poor care or being denied care (Nelson, 1997; James and Platzer, 1999); fear of being treated for homosexuality as a pathology, particularly if the individual is anxious or depressed (Robertson, 1997); and for lesbians, fear that they may lose custody of a child or have difficulties arranging child care (Hall, 1994). Such concerns are due to a perceived lack of understanding of the implications of an 'other' lifestyle among healthcare workers. Equally, an individual choosing not to disclose must maintain a level of deception and, as a result, may receive inappropriate health care or information. As an example, Bird (1999) reports how lesbians and gay men disabled with multiple sclerosis may receive care in a residential home where homophobia can lead to isolation, which in turn can be a cause for depression. For transgendered persons, there may be issues around providing care in a male or female setting.

While heterosexual relationships are upheld by recognised familial, legal and institutional structures, lesbians, gay men and transgendered persons do not benefit from this same protection. This position can increase social isolation, when a partner or significant person is not acknowledged or included because they are not 'family' (Stevens, 1992; Platzer, 1993) and can alienate individuals from the healthcare process — a disempowering experience. It can leave the individuals without self-validation and positive connections (Hall, 1999), factors that may account for increased risk of depression and suicide among lesbian and gay men (Nelson, 1994; Nelson, 1997; Shelby, 1999; Hall, 1999).

This can be the cost of feeling silenced by a heterosexist system. As Lorde declares:

> *I wanted to talk to a lesbian, to sit down and start from a common language, no matter how diverse. I wanted to share dyke-insight, so to speak.*

(Lorde, 1980, p. 41)

In this particular situation, Audre Lorde, a black lesbian, felt alienated by advice given about the need for a prosthesis following mastectomy. She did not want a prosthesis but was told that she should have one to look good as a woman and that not to have a prosthesis would be bad for staff morale. Her primary concerns were about her personal survival and control over her life, not about sex role stereotypes for women. Engaging in inappropriate health care can have very negative effects. James and Platzer (1999) in their focus group research with British lesbians and gay men heard how individuals felt unsafe, uncomfortable and anxious about receiving health care. For some, this results in direct avoidance of health care (Stevens, 1994; Nelson, 1997; James and Platzer, 1999) with consequential deteriorating health, while others who do engage, have experiences of rough handling and sexual abuse by healthcare workers (James and Platzer, 1999).

Considering these reported experiences, it becomes easier to understand why some lesbians, gay men and transgendered persons may be very reluctant to engage in the healthcare process. It also goes some way in explaining the increased risk of depression and suicide among these groups of people and the reported high incidence of alcohol and drug use (Nelson, 1994; Hobbs, 1994; Ryan *et al*, 1998; Meese, 1997; Selby, 1999). Living in a stigmatising society has a direct impact on health needs and healthcare experiences, and it has been suggested that negative healthcare experiences result in reduced trust in healthcare workers generally (Caress *et al*, 1998).

For many lesbians, gay men and transgendered persons, engaging in the healthcare process is a negative experience. There are some reported positive interactions and these focus on good communication, acceptance of the individual's sexual orientation in a matter of fact manner, respect and inclusion of an identified partner/family, sensitivity and compassion and being nursed by lesbians and gay men (Stevens, 1994; James and Platzer, 1999). These elements should be recognised and built upon in any attempt to empower lesbians, gay men and transgendered individuals to participate in healthcare provision.

Challenging heterosexism in health care: Empowering lesbians, gay men and transgendered individuals

The movement within healthcare provision that is centralising the user means that:

> *Health service staff need to understand that empowerment
> of service users should not be viewed as something they
> can choose to bestow or withhold.*

(Iskander, 1999, p. 31)

The implicit heterosexism in the services, once highlighted, cannot be ignored and leaves us with a moral obligation to pay attention to the needs and experiences of those alienated through their sexuality (James and Platzer, 1999). The necessity for this is confirmed by the fact that the National Institute For Clinical Effectiveness (NICE) insists that users' experiences should provide a central measurement for effectiveness within the NHS. Looking at the experiences of lesbians, gay men and transgendered persons in this chapter shows that levels of effectiveness of care are very low for these groups and that healthcare workers feel inadequately trained in issues of sexuality (Nerdahl *et al*, 1999). How can services be improved and lesbians, gay men and transgendered individuals be empowered to participate in healthcare processes?

It is possible to consider three main arenas for action that may help to uncover heterosexism and homophobia while maintaining at least some centrality and providing empowerment for the lesbians, gay men and transgendered user. These arenas are:

- purchasers/providers
- practice settings
- academic settings.

Purchasers/providers of services

These organisations should engage in outreach work (Kreiss and Patterson, 1997) to identify local groups representing lesbians, gay men and transgendered persons. This would be a bridge-building exercise that would then enable liaison between user representatives and purchasers/providers. There is a need to create at this level an environment that encourages participation by alienated or stigmatised groups. Contact should be initiated with such groups as the Beaumont Society (for transgendered persons) and lesbian and gay men's groups. Lesbians, gay men and transgendered individuals need to be made visible within local populations and their healthcare needs acknowledged. It is highly likely that there will be resistance to such work, as it seems that many people believe that lesbians, gay men and transgendered people now 'have it easy', with high profile public individuals being openly gay or lesbian and challenging rigid gender stereotypes. However, resistance can be countered by the described need to engage users in the planning and organising of healthcare services.

Practice settings

Empowerment for lesbians, gay men and transgendered persons may be initiated by creating an environment that is not heterosexual specific. The Sarah Bernhardt Clinic for lesbians is a good example of a very specific healthcare practice setting. This may more generally be achieved through inclusive assessment procedures that ask each individual what their sexual orientation is (Ryan, 1998). This helps to create a matter of fact feeling about sexuality and enables subsequent questions and information to be appropriate to the individual. (There is a danger that information may be withheld as being inappropriate, for example, in identifying sexual health needs it should not be assumed that gay men never have sexual intercourse with women.) When seeking information about relationships, terms such as wife or husband should not be used until they have been identified by the user. This allows for non-heterosexist terms like partner or significant person to be employed. Language needs to be inclusive (Nelson, 1997; Godfrey, 1999) so that individuals may feel in charge and can choose to disclose their sexuality or not. Newberry (1996) argues that healthcare workers should not try to impose a heterosexual model of relationships onto gay men and Meese (1997) specifically identifies the central role of the general practitioner in meeting the healthcare needs of the transgendered person.

Visibility for lesbians, gay men and transgendered persons may be increased by having relevant health literature displayed. A clear example is seen in HIV literature which is directed at specific target groups, so that the literature for lesbians is different from that for heterosexual women. Visibility within the environment can help to create a feeling of confirmation (Hall, 1999) which needs to be supported by staff understanding of issues pertinent to lesbians, gay men and transgendered individuals. Healthcare workers need to understand and acknowledge how illness may affect the individual and their lifestyle (Bird, 1999) in order to create a supportive environment that can enable participation in the healthcare process. This should be coupled with the recognition of the limitations of the service (Bird, 1999). For example, an older person requiring residential care is unlikely to find a 'gay friendly' home or one where cross-dressing would be acceptable — perhaps an issue for purchasers/providers to consider. O'Connor *et al* (1999) describes this clearly:

Patients need to comprehend the options and the outcomes in order to consider and communicate the personal value they place on the benefits versus the harms.

(O'Connor *et al*, 1999, p. 733)

These authors fail to recognise that sexual orientation may have a bearing on the effectiveness of the service, although they acknowledge the impact of age, sex and ethnicity. Details of local and national organisations offering support to lesbians, gay men and transgendered persons should be displayed to enable individuals to seek appropriate help if needed. Healthcare workers should be aware of these resources (Ryan, 1998; Shelby, 1999; Godfrey, 1999) so that they may provide information as required. The importance of visibility is emphasised by Whittle (1998) who argues that for transgendered persons, there is empowerment through not attempting to be invisible and that there is a movement within the transgendered community to redefine the medical processes of transgender. This visibility and authenticity is promoted through global networking via the Internet. Healthcare workers needs to be aware of this positive and confirming resource for transgendered people.

Literature reveals that the overall demeanour of healthcare workers can have a major impact on lesbians, gay men and transgendered users. It is essential to create a sense of safety, ensure confidentiality and provide compassionate, empathic care (Whittle, 1998; Godfrey, 1999). Lesbians, gay men and transgendered health workers may provide additional support if they feel able to 'come out', as one of the reported positive experiences was being cared for by people of a similar orientation. Indeed, this type of interaction may be empowering for user and worker alike.

Robertson (1997) argues that mental health nurses, in particular, need a good understanding of issues relating to gay men. This is important when symptoms of mental distress relate to living in a stigmatising society and should be expanded to mental health workers appreciating factors relating to the lives of lesbians, gay men and transgendered persons, the 'outsider within' perspective. Mental health users need to be encouraged into being involved in decisions that affect their care for this can have a profound effect, as reported by one service user:

It's given me a life and without it I wouldn't have dreamed
of doing half the things I do now. It's given me confidence,
assurance.

(Barnes *et al*, 1999, p. 94)

Essential practices that empower lesbians, gay men and transgendered users include centralising the individual, recognising and respecting their uniqueness — valuing difference. Fear comes through ignorance; healthcare workers have a personal and professional responsibility to educate and inform themselves. As Shelby identified:

Widespread ignorance and discrimination are the primary
causes of most of the health issues facing gay, lesbian and
bisexual youth.

(Shelby, 1999, p. 29).

It does not demand much imagination to see how this can be applied to older gay men, lesbians, bisexuals and transgendered persons when reflecting on the evidence given in this chapter.

The academic setting

The identification of heterosexism underpinning healthcare services and the reported experiences of lesbians, gay men and transgendered users reveals the major role that education has to play in the process of empowering the identified groups to participation. The 'outsider within' perspective reveals anomalies in an NHS which is supposedly centralising the users of the service. James and Platzer (1999) encountered real funding problems for research that would expose the silencing and prejudice of a section of the population. There may be an increased tolerance of lesbians, gay men and transgendered persons in society but if that does not transpose to positive action it is worthless. Raymond wrote in 1980 (p. 176):

Tolerance can be oppressive... functioning as sympathy
for the oppressed,

and this may describe the current position. Sympathy is not useful: attitudinal and behavioural change and a willingness to understand is required before empowerment and participation can be achieved. Research in this area needs active support, particularly in today's setting of evidence-based practice. Increased research would provide further evidence of healthcare experiences and needs of lesbians, gay men and transgendered users and would facilitate the incorporation of this knowledge in the day-to-day teaching of all healthcare workers. Sexual orientation is both a personal and a political agenda. Education needs to cover sex role stereotyping and the rigid gendering within society, institutionalised heterosexism, the evolvement of sexual identity and its impact on lifestyle, the process of 'coming out' and the dynamics of same sex families, as well as close inspection of personal attitudes and beliefs of healthcare workers. Healthcare workers need to be made aware of local and national resources and to recognise that lesbians, gay men and transgendered persons do not have the same familial, social, legal support and protection that heterosexuals enjoy. This education needs to be provided with sensitivity and respect for these groups of people who live, by necessity, on the edges of acceptability. It is no easy task because of the dominant discourses that pervade our thinking, speaking and experiencing. Challenging and deconstructing these discourses cause anxiety and discomfort, but this is surely a small price to pay if the result is more effective health care for lesbians, gay men and transgendered persons, and a health care that includes empowerment and participation.

Within this chapter I have attempted to consider ways in which specific groups marginalised within society may be heard and centralised in the healthcare process. The 'outsider within' perspective enables us to reflect on processes that we may take for granted as being effective, and allows us to question time-honoured beliefs and practices as we consider them from an alternative viewpoint. I have identified some of the deleterious effects of living with stigma and prejudice and highlighted some means of overcoming institutionalised oppressive practices. Perhaps the biggest question to be raised from this work is how best to challenge a system where heterosexism is so imbued, it is often not even recognised? Hope is essential in this task and is described by Hall (1999) as:

> ... *a liberation based aspect of health that enhances the authenticity of relations and fuels personal and collective empowerment.*

> (Hall, 1999, p. 100)

Key points

⌘ The care and treatment of people who are lesbian or gay is often adversely affected by assumptions that 'to be heterosexual is the normal, proper and fixed sexual identity'.

⌘ The social reality of lesbian, gay and transgendered individuals is unacknowledged, both in health services and in political, economic and other social systems. However, participants of various organisations, as 'outsiders within', have promulgated social realities which challenge heterosexism.

⌘ Understanding the social realities of lesbian, gay and transgendered people can enable health services to more effectively meet their needs.

⌘ Stigmatisation and exclusion from health services can affect these individuals' self-esteem and self-worth, and the extent to which they feel valued and accepted. Transgendered people often face particular rejection. Considerable stress, ill health and internalised homophobia may result from stigmatisation in wider society, attempts to 'pass', and struggles for self-acceptance.

⌘ Assessment and care of clients often include assumptions that they are heterosexual or have a 'static gender identity'. Lack of understanding can contribute to isolation, alienation and stereotyping in health services and in wider society.

⌘ Providing a voice is the basis of empowerment for lesbian, gay and transgendered individuals. It is important that their perspectives are reflected in health service practice and information; research and its funding; and purchasers' and providers' attempts to enable participation.

⌘ Good practice includes assessment and care which is sensitive to the needs and experiences of lesbian, gay and transgendered people and their partners; visible health literature which confirms their identity; recognition of the limitations of services; ensuring confidentiality; and the provision of 'compassionate, empathic care' that values the individual. Relevant staff education and information are important.

Jane Godfrey

References

Adam J (1995) Caring for the 'new' family in palliative care. *Br J Nurs* **4**(21): 1253–71

Bailey ME (1993) Foucauldian feminism: contesting bodies, sexuality and identity. In: Ramazanaglu C *Up against Foucault. Explorations of some tensions between Foucault and feminism*. Routledge, London

Barnes M (1999) *Unequal partners*. The Policy Press, Bristol

Bird D (1999) Get glammed up. *Nurs Standard* **13**(30): 20

Cahill J (1988) Patient participation — a review of the literature. *J Clin Nurs* **7**: 119–28

Cain M (1993) Foucault, feminism and feeling. What Foucault can and cannot contribute to feminist epistemology. In: Ramazanaglu C *Up Against Foucault. Explorations of some tensions between Foucault and feminism*. Routledge, London.

Caress A, Luker KA, Ackrill P (1998) Patient sensitive treatment decision making? Preferences and perceptions in a sample of renal patients. *NT Res* **3**(5): 364–72

Collins PH (1991) *Black Feminist Thought. Knowledge, consciousness and the politics of empowerment*. Routledge, London

Department of Health (1991) *The Patient's Charter*. DoH, London

Department of Health (1994) *Working in Partnership*. DoH, London

Department of Health (1997) *The new NHS — modern, dependable*. The Stationery Office, London

Diva (2000) *Lesbian life and style*. April: 29–30

Foucault M (1987) *The History of Sexuality*. Penguin, London

Fraher T, Limpinnian M (1999) User empowerment within mental health nursing. In: Wilkinson G, Miers M, eds. *Power and Nursing Practice*. Macmillan, Basingstoke

Godfrey J (1999) Empowerment through sexuality. In: Wilkinson G, Miers M, eds. *Power and Nursing Practice*. Macmillan, Basingstoke

Gray P, Kramer M, Minick P, McGehee L, Thomas D, Greiner D (1996) Heterosexism in nursing education. *J Nurse Educ* **35**(5): 204–10

Hall JM (1994) Lesbians recovering from alcohol problems: an ethnographic study of health care experiences. *Nurs Res* July/August: 238–44.

Hall JM (1999) Marginalisation revisited: critical, postmodern and liberation perspectives. *Adv Nurs Science*, December: 88–102

Hickey G, Kipping C (1998) Exploring the concept of user involvement in mental health through a participatory continuum. *J Clinic Nurs* **7**: 83–8

Hugman R (1991) *Power in Caring Professionals*. Macmillan, London

Illich I (1976) *Medical Nemesis. The appropriation of health*. Pantheon, New York

Iskander R (1999) Listen and learn. *Nurs Times* **95**(13): 30–1

James T, Platzer H (1999) Ethical considerations in qualitative research with vulnerable groups: exploring lesbians' and gay men's experiences of health care — a personal perspective. *Nurs Ethics* **6**(1): 75–81

Jones A (1988) Nothing gay about bereavement. *Nurs Times* **84**(23): 55–7

Kreiss JL, Patterson DL (1997) Psychosocial issues in primary care of lesbians, gays, bisexuals and transgender youth. *J Pediatr Health Care* **11**(16): 266–74

Lorde A (1980) *The Cancer Journals*. Sheba Feminist Publishers, London

Loulan J (1984) *Lesbian Sex*. Spinsters. Aunt Lute. San Francisco

Lynch MA (1993) When the patient is also a lesbian. Association for Women's Health, Obstetric and Neonatal Nurses (AWONNS). Clinical Issues. *Perinatal Women's Health* **4**(2) 196–202

Mahoney C (1999) Mothers of contention. *Nurs Times* **95**(31): 12, 13

McHale A (1996) Risk reduction strategies in the control of AIDS. *Professional Nurse* **11**: 731–3

Meese P (1997) The role of the general practitioner in the care of the transgendered patient. *Venereology* **10**(3): 154–7

Nelson JA (1994) Comment on special issue on adolescence. *Am Psychologist*, June: 523–4

Nelson JA (1997) Gay, lesbian and bisexual adolescents: providing esteem enhancing care to a battered population. *Nurse Pract* **22**(2): 94, 99, 103, 106, 109

Nemoto T, Luke D, Mamo L, Ching A, Patria J (1999) HIV risk behaviors among male to female transgenders in comparison with homosexual or bisexual males and heterosexual females. *AIDS Care* **11**(13): 297–312

Nerdhal P, Berglund D, Beavinger LH, Saewyc E, Ireland M, Evans T (1999) New challenges, new answers: pediatric nurse practitioners and the care of adolescents. *J Pediatr Health Care* **13**(4):183–90

Newberry D (1996) Exploring gay relationships. *Nurs Standard* **10**(16): 54–6

O'Connor AM, Rostom A, Fiset V, Tetro J, Entwistle V, Llewellyn-Thomas H, Holmes-Rovner M, Barry M, Jones J (1999) Decision aids for patients facing health treatment or screening decisions: systematic review. *Br Med J* **319**: 731–4

Platzer H (1993) Nursing care of gay and lesbian patients. *Nurs Standard* **7**(17): 34–7

Ranade W (1997) *A Future for the NHS? Health Care For The Millennium.* 2nd edn. Longman, London

Raymond JG (1980) *The Transsexual Empire.* The Women's Press, London

Rickford F (1995) Battle lines. *Community Care*, 5–11 August: 12

Robertson AE (1997) The mental health experiences of gay men: a research study exploring gay men's health needs. *J Psychiatr Mental Health Nurs* **5**: 33–40

Ryan C, Futterman D, Stine K (1998) Helping our hidden youth. *Am J Nurs* **98**(12): 37–41

Shelby P (1999) Isolated and invisible. Gay, lesbian and bisexual youth. *Can Youth*, April: 27–30

Soper K (1993) Productive contradictions. In: Ramazanoglu C *Up Against Foucault. Explorations of some tensions between foucault and feminism.* Routledge, London

Stevens PE, Hall JM (1988) Stigma, health beliefs and experiences with health care in lesbian women. *Image J Nurs Scholarship* **20**(2): 69–73

Stevens PE (1992) Lesbian health care research: a review of the literature from 1970–1990. *Health Care for Women International* **13**(2): 91–120

Stevens PE (1994) Lesbians' health-related experience of care and non care. *Western J Nurs Res* **16**(6): 639–59

Valios N (1999) Extending the family. *Community Care*, 5–11 August: 12

Weeks J (1986) *Sexuality.* Routledge, London

Weeks J (1991) *Against Nature.* Rivers Oram Press, London

Whittle S (1998) The trans-cyberian mail way. *Social and Legal Studies* **7**(3): 391–408. Sage, London

7

A question of 'choices and space': gay, lesbian and transgender services in North Warwickshire

Paul Fitzgerald

This chapter will highlight the work of North Warwickshire NHS Trust in addressing the issues of the mental health needs of those gay, lesbian and transgender people who live in and around North Warwickshire. Although based on mental health need, the service delivery takes place across both mental health day services and sexual health services for young people.

In 1991, North Warwickshire Health Promotion Service made a bid to the Regional NHS Executive to develop sexual health services for young people in Nuneaton and Bedworth.

A development bid of £56,000 was given to 'do something about teenage pregnancy'. The 1990 census had highlighted the high rate of teenage pregnancy in this county. From this vague and humble beginning the 'health store' service began.

Health store has developed a range of sexual health services for young people under twenty-five and is seen both locally and nationally as a service of excellence. As part of the development of the health store service, a needs assessment analysis was undertaken and Public Health Medicine were asked to process it. It became apparent that health services for young people across the board were sorely lacking. The services that existed had not always addressed the specific problems which prevent young people from accessing services. Health store therefore developed as a holistic health and welfare advice service, trying to meet the health needs of young people across a range of areas, which include sexual health and mental health (NHS Management Executive, 1992).

Joint working with local further education college

Early in 1992, an outreach service of health store began at North Warwickshire College of Further Education. Services provided included free condoms, pregnancy testing, general health advice and information and counselling on sexual health issues. Almost immediately more enquiries for counselling were received than could be delivered (Health Store, Contract Monitoring 1992, April–September).

Several of those initial enquiries were from students who presented as gay or lesbian and who needed support for a variety of reasons.

Working closely with the college student liaison team, we developed the 'pink triangle' support group and agreed to meet weekly in a porta-cabin on the college site. Despite some 'sassy' publicity and knowing we already had several contacts with students, we were naively surprised when only two people attended. Further discussion revealed that the gay and lesbian students felt too exposed to attend a visible group on the college campus, and this seemingly negative beginning, gave them the chance to raise some issues about homophobic bullying.

Health store staff and the college student liaison team, working closely with the students already identified, relaunched the support group off campus.

Health store runs its service from a community centre in the middle of Nuneaton. The centre is called 'Hatters Space' (it was originally part of a local hat factory) and is conveniently close to both train and bus stations. It was felt that this site would be a more suitable and safe space, and so the group began.

Focus and participation

The young clients identified three clear objectives for the group:

1. A place to meet other young people of the same sexual orientation, and to attend social events.
2. A safe place to discuss and share information about any difficulties that arise as a result of their sexuality.
3. An opportunity to access one-to-one support from health professionals.

Promotion and advertising

Remaining clear about the concerns that the young students had identified in terms of safety, we advertised the group with telephone contact numbers only.

Training was given to reception staff who might be the first contact when a young person made the initial call.

We arranged a meeting place just a few minutes away from the centre and organised for a worker and an existing member to meet prospective new members and to escort them to the group; this achieved two things:

1. It provided an opportunity for screening to ensure prospective members are genuine.
2. It eased entry to the group by ensuring that no one has to walk in on their own.

Flyers and posters were distributed around the college campus, local libraries and youth centres. Information was sent to social work teams, GP practices and the adolescent mental health service.

The group met successfully in this form for a period of two years. The number of young people attending the group at any one time was fairly small, (average age sixteen), a maximum of eleven by April 1994. However, for those young people who attended, the value of the support they received was immeasurable. As individuals they gained great support from each other.

Those individuals who needed more support had direct access to a counsellor.

The group spent quite a lot of time addressing safer sex issues:

- negotiating safer sex
- HIV and testing
- staying safe 'on the scene'.

By September 1994, some of the original members had moved on, some to university or to employment, and left the group because of relationships ending. Staff also changed as people moved on into new posts.

Difficulties, errors made, lessons learnt

During that period the contract for direct work in the HIV field rested with the HIV network and its sub-groups (later to become Terence Higgins Trust West Midlands and now THT Lighthouse West Midlands).

The organisations at that time were not sufficiently funded to do direct work across the whole of Warwickshire, and focused their work in Coventry, with some joint working with health promotion departments across the county.

Professionals across different settings work in vastly different ways and priorities for voluntary sector organisations, statutory organisations, and others can be widely different.

Organisations found themselves competing for the same budgets, and individuals working in the sexual health field held finely guarded opinions as to the best way to provide services.

Although joint meetings were held and differences aired, successful joint working did not happen at that time.

The voluntary sector agencies felt that SPACE should have been a service of their organisation, although because of the lack of targeted funds they could not work in this district. There was also some criticism of some of the support staff of SPACE, for although properly qualified and experienced, not all support staff were gay or lesbian and were therefore not seen to be suitable role models. Some young clients as they matured moved between the SPACE group in Nuneaton and the support group run by the network in Coventry. This group is called GYGL (Godiva young gay and lesbians) and it is felt that both groups meet a need, and do not need to compete with one another.

Much of the friction between organisations has been resolved over time, but developments may have been easier if countywide strategies had been in place, so that everyone felt their work was valued. Individuals and groups could have then perceived themselves as part of the whole structure, rather than an isolated and unconnected island. A holistic approach is fine, but it is impossible to provide everything for everyone on a fixed budget.

SPACE continued to provide services for young people but in a much-reduced way until April 1998.

SPACE — the re-launch

By 1999, new health promotion specialists were in post with a specific interest in supporting the SPACE group.

Also North Warwickshire NHS Community Trust was looking at its equal opportunities policy and addressing gaps in its delivery of sexuality support, and promoted a mental health services equality initiative to address the mental health needs of people who are gay, lesbian, bisexual or transgender.

Mental health services have historically offered a poor service to people who do not define themselves as heterosexual or who have issues around gender identity. The response more often than not has been one of anthologising difference and, until relatively recently, offering treatment aimed at helping the person to be 'normal'.

Attitudes are more enlightened now but, even though homosexuality is no longer seen as an illness in its own right, there is very little acknowledgement of the impact of society's prejudice and hostility on the mental health of people who are gay, lesbian, bisexual or transgender. This lack of acknowledgement can make it very difficult for someone to talk openly about their sexual or gender identity in the course of treatment for mental illness. This, of course, disempowers those individuals whose denial of who they are remains secret. As a direct consequence, whatever treatment is given, it risks falling rather wide of the mark.

> The concept behind SPACE is to enable and empower gay, lesbian and bisexual young people to develop self-esteem and a positive attitude to both themselves and their sexuality. As we live in a predominantly heterosexual society, young people may find identifying with themselves extremely difficult and stressful. Living up to heterosexual values commonly held by peers, friends, parents and family is often impossible.
>
> SPACE aims to allow young gay, lesbian and bisexual people the time and place to be open with themselves and others.
>
> SPACE where no one has gone before.

Claire Cahill, Student liaison officer,
North Warwickshire and Hinckley College

In August 1997, North Warwickshire NHS Trust piloted a post targeted at service users who were identified as gay, lesbian, bisexual or transgender, and ran two sessions a week. The post-holder was already employed as a counsellor with the trust and was out as a gay. The take up for the initiative was immediate and on the strength of this initial pilot, in October 1999, the post was made full-time.

CHOICES — committed to equality

Developed in 1999, the CHOICES initiative has been developed to provide a range of services to individuals who identify as gay, lesbian, bisexual and transgender. Its aims are:

- to raise awareness of the mental health needs of people who are gay, lesbian, bisexual and transgender and to seek to address those needs
- to provide high quality services to promote the changing of attitudes towards difference in society
- to promote equal opportunities and speak up for social injustices
- to challenge oppression, discrimination and prejudice.

The initiative also provides a counselling service, advocacy, advice and information support groups for young people and older adults.

This service provision aims to empower service users who in the past had no appropriate provision aimed specifically at their needs.

A selection of case histories

Although I had been out and living openly with my male partner, this was never acknowledged by the mental health professionals. Whenever I became ill my partner had to telephone my father to find out what was happening. They never once involved my partner in my case, he did not exist as a real member of my family. This added to my sense of not being normal and that my mental health was somehow linked to my sexuality and this was the problem.

At the moment I am working through my feelings with my counsellor, to deal with my hurt and anger towards mental health professionals who should have known better.

Steve/'manic depressive'

Therapy has enabled me to learn about who I am, what I am and, most importantly, how to become more assertive in my dealings with healthcare professionals. I am now able to challenge my psychiatrist/ nursing staff and my therapist if I feel I am being treated unfairly.

Carl/CHOICES group member

Being a lesbian was so alien to me that I tried to hide my true self for many years, this resulted in trying to end my life on several occasions. When I told my community psychiatric nurse what the problem was she put me in touch with the CHOICES group. This has been a lifesaver — literally! I feel more confident and proud of myself for the first time in my life.

Kym/CHOICES group member

I never told anyone about my sexual preference for twenty years, in the end I was asked to fill in a form/questionnaire and when asked what the overriding problems were I put down dealing with my sexuality.

For two weeks I worried constantly about the reaction from the psychologist. When we did meet, he was great. He reassured me and told me about the services that were available locally and put me in touch with Paul. I have not looked back since.

Kevin/CHOICES group member

Being married with three children and hiding my sexuality is and has been hard work. I felt totally disempowered to do anything about my situation and became ill. The community psychiatric nurse kept on dropping hints about sexuality (she has told me since, she had discussed my case with a gay worker) and in the end I told her about myself. The relief was enormous. I found acceptance, support and encouragement.

Sue/'in therapy'

A friend of Dorothy's

My name is Richard. I've been going to the Nuneaton gay and lesbian social group for about a year and a bit. The group has helped me tremendously over the past year. I didn't even dream of coming out; a year ago I had not even dealt with the fact in my own mind. I felt isolated, uncertain of my future, scared of what people would think, afraid of being gay. I needed someone who would understand me (sometimes better than myself) who could relate to the torment I'm going through. I needed someone who could help me find my way through this nightmare. I had to tell someone I could trust. When I did, it felt as though a ton of bricks had been lifted from my shoulders.

Apart from finding a valuable support network, I found a true, honest friend. The group has been a milestone of help and support, not only by helping me feel comfortable and confident about my sexuality, but also by discussing other personal issues like college and career development. The group has given me a new direction in life, to know that you are not the only one.

Thinking back to when I was at school, the only reason I didn't come out in my final years was because I was afraid of people's reactions, and how they would treat me. I realise now through the knowledge the group has given me, that I had internalised homophobia. I was afraid because society made me afraid. I grew up in a society where I was not given any positive images of homosexuality, or never taught or discussed the issue at school. This is where the apathy starts, you grow up believing the things that the people you look up to, tell you, that being a queer is wrong and AIDS is the cure. You get the impression that all gays are sex mad, outrageous drama queens, and they all float about in their own little fairy-like worlds bonking each other senseless.

Myths and misconceptions that if you hang around with gay people you will somehow by magic end up being one, or that you are the son of Satan. That he can't be a queer he's married and got two kids, what garbage people think. But people only think these zany conceptions because of the lack of information available and the fact that it is far easier to victimise and criticise us, than look at us in a more positive manner. Ominously, like so many groups in society, we are a minority in a majority but as soon as the majority realise we are just like them (well almost) and all we want is the same opportunities and quality of life as them.

I find it disheartening that people can treat us as the scum of the earth, just because of our sexual preference. What gives them the right? I didn't choose to be gay, I was born like it, but... I doubt we will ever be fully accepted into society, and seen as normal human beings because, sadly, society and people has always needed its loathed scapegoats and there is little finesse in its methods for showing it. The bounty for such prejudice and hatred started from the Bible. Its instinctive dislike of homosexuals has resulted from decades into centuries of fear and contempt played upon by religious homophobes. In one breath they speak of loving thy neighbour, in another of the evil of homosexuality. It is narrow-minded bigots like these that have spread the fear and hatred towards not just gay people, but any group in society. Hatred and bigotry will always remain regardless what positive images and arguments are put forward. What would it take to change people's minds about us so called bum bandits? If Princess Diana couldn't do it by holding the hands of people with AIDS then I doubt that even a bastion of respectability could do it.

Being gay is only a small part of my life but one of the most important parts. Therefore, it is paramount that I feel comfortable and confident about being gay. Otherwise I am open to homophobic slander and remarks and this weakens you as an individual. That's when other areas of your life begin to be affected. Given the choice now, whether to be gay or straight, I would without hesitation choose to be gay. As you gain confidence and self-esteem you realise that being gay is not your problem, it's theirs.

My advice:

Take time to think? — give yourself time to reflect. Deciding that you might be or are gay is one of the hardest things you can do as an individual. You feel afraid, mixed up, frustrated, you want answers to why you feel this way.

Why me? — you ask yourself, why the hell me? Life would be far more simple and less complex if I did not feel this way.

Accepting it — you are not on your own, thousands of people feel the same way as you and there are people who can help.

Give yourself time! — take one day at a time and don't be hard on yourself, let the answers come to you, give yourself space.

First step — once you have made the first move to get in contact with a group, you will be amazed how much it will help. Meeting new people getting involved makes a difference.

Richard/CHOICES group member

Although I had been 'out' to my close friends for some time, I wasn't particularly self-confident about my sexuality and was still quite worried about how people would react to my being gay. Coming to 'SPACE' helped to change that, by meeting other people who felt the same as me, I really felt a sense of belonging. Having a space to talk about any problems I might have, being able to meet people who were also gay, and confident about that. SPACE has really changed my outlook to life and to myself.

Kevin (aged seventeen) SPACE member 1995–1997

Having been in boarding school (and all boys) and then joining college, having no one to turn too, and living in an army environment, counsellors at college helped me and enhanced my courage to come out in public. Joining a gay and lesbian group called 'SPACE' was or is an excellent idea, especially now people from college know me as a person rather than a label. It's a good place to get away and be you and chat about anything and organising outings for the group to join in and getting to know other groups around the country. So, yes, 'SPACE' is a great place to be yourself, I've done it, so can you!

Scott (art and design student, aged eighteen)
SPACE member 1994–1996

Benefits and outcomes

❖ Improvement in the mental health of the service users included in this work has been significant. Increased self-confidence has been a part of this process to the extent that several members of the support group played an active part in a seminar on mental health and sexual identity, which was held by the trust in 1999.

❖ Feedback from staff has been positive in that the availability of this resource has enabled staff to have a greater clarity in their clinical interventions with service users.

❖ Although there have been some difficulties reflecting the homophobic attitudes which exist in society, these have been minor and have been far outweighed by the positive response from staff and service users.

- Transgender work brings its own set of issues. Although there was no anticipation of significant numbers, in fact the project did not originally include this brief — offering this service has uncovered an unmet need.
- Although there is a knowledge base on transgender issues, it is not widely shared or discussed. Levels of awareness in society and among mental health professionals are variable. People wishing to, or in the process of reassessing their gender encounter varying levels of understanding and sensitivity.
- The CHOICES project offers both a counselling and liaison role and has been broadly welcomed as a model of good practice.

Key points

- Young people with sexual orientation issues need a safe place to discuss and share information, opportunities to access one-to-one support from health professionals and a protected place to meet other young people of the same focus.
- Professionals across different settings work in vastly different ways and priorities for voluntary sector organisations, statutory organizations, and others can be widely different. When different organisations find themselves competing for the same budgets, the target groups suffer.
- People wishing to, or in the process of reassessing their gender, encounter varying levels of understanding and sensitivity as levels of awareness and prejudice in society and among professionals are variable.
- Gay affirmation therapy is not an independent system of therapy. It represents a special range of psychological knowledge which challenges the traditional view that homosexual desire and fixed homosexual orientations are pathological.
- One-to-one support from health professionals has seen significant improvements in the mental health of the service users.

References

Health Store (1992) *Contract Monitoring* (April – September) North Warwickshire NHS Trust. Nuneaton

NHS Management Executive (1992) *Guidelines for Reviewing Family Planning Services*. Criteria one — range of provision. HMSO, London

8

Drumming on the sidelines: a user experience of involvement in local strategic planning

Anonymous

I had apparently lost out in the roulette of birth: parental alcoholism, poverty and deprivation. I occasionally suffered malnutrition throughout childhood and was on the receiving end of various forms of abuse at home and elsewhere. Ativan (now known to be an addictive substance) became the first 'cure' for my distress at the age of thirteen. It worked so well, I had a schizophrenia diagnosis at the age of nineteen and had progressed onto Largactil, Melleril and other major tranquillisers.

I was an out-patient mostly, turning up at least once a week at the out-patient clinic for almost seven years. I have vague memories of a violent sectioning. To this day, I have no idea of my term on the lock-up ward. I was received at hospital, became very aggressive at the bureaucratic delays, was restrained and then 'Goodnight, goodnight, Thorazine'.

Eventually I met a psychiatrist at out-patients, who knew that my days of sleep and shakes on major tranquillisers were over. She had a warped belief that I might learn to cope and begin self-helping without psychiatry. I knew she was mad, as the socially endorsed knowledge of previous professional input had convinced me of the permanency of my situation. Her advanced intuition proved correct, despite majority opinion. Some years later, I joined a mental health user group, having in the meantime emigrated from Ireland to England.

My first experience of mental health strategic management was when I was invited by my housing support worker to become a management committee member of a local MIND in 1991. This was an honour, as I had an established reputation for not being a very subservient or compliant resident of their group homes. Despite my self-perceived lack of qualification, I was co-opted and elected at the next annual general meeting. Although there were some protracted disagreements at long arduous committee meetings, my teeth were cut.

In general, my work and time were respected and my input as an Irish person and a service user was valued. Though Irish people constituted a major segment of the local population, it was unusual locally to have Irish input at management level, especially of the unprivileged variety. Irish people are predominantly white and deemed adequately represented by 'White-UKs' at health strategic levels in England.

I could never quite follow the logic of this. Such assumptions have always appeared to me as an awkward-to-challenge excuse for exclusion and a means of diluting Irish into English health experience, despite evidence of Irish over-representations in ill-health and disadvantage statistics.

Shortly after my term with MIND, I was co-opted onto management of the locally formed mental health service user group. Soon, I was formally invited to attend the local council's disability sub-committee as a non-voting user participant. Under instruction from the local user group, I lobbied, with some grounds for success, to have 'people with mental health difficulties' acknowledged as a distinct grouping on the council's equal opportunity policy.

On the day of the sub-committee debate, I was shattered to hear a prominent councillor opine: 'We do not want these mentally subnormal people on our equal opportunity policy.' Disappointingly, his comment did not provoke any challenge or response from those that mattered. The motion was moved to another committee and became lost in the bureaucratic void.

After my year (four meetings!) watching the disability sub-committee talk a lot of non-innovation, I was voted by the local user group onto the newly set-up mental health strategy group. This group consisted of local and health authority officials, as well as the chief officer of the local community health council, my nervy self and one other user group representative, who resigned very quickly. After this resignation, I was the only member to live locally; the other members contentedly commuting to our unpopular borough. There was no black representation, despite the borough having one of the highest percentages of black minorities in the UK.

This group was much more pro-active than the council sub-committee referred to previously, meeting very regularly and setting up working groups to report back to the main group. The chair of the group was a health authority official. All seemed anxious to please him and not to rock too many boats. It seemed to me that careers were very important indeed and 'on-the-line' if a dissident opinion was expressed. The world of health administration in England is obviously small and requires sacrifices of silence for personal advancement.

I became a prized puppet of other members of the group, who fed me discrediting information on each other to disturb the false 'equilibrium'. Many important meetings were disrupted with my 'is-it-true-that' point scoring interrogation of various other members. I became a willing (though unknowing at first) pawn in a strategic pique and power game played out between the health and local authorities, and also between individuals within each authority.

The user agenda for the strategy was known, several worthwhile local consultations having taken place. The health and social care professionals knew exactly which buttons to push before a meeting to gain maximum vocal tirades from me to the chair and other individuals. It took me some time to realise that while I was in confrontation, I was not pushing the user agenda and the subjective strategy of the chair was merrily trundling forward, without challenge.

Another difficulty was language. Research and briefing papers and reports were all couched in academic language. The draft strategy itself was almost a foreign tongue to the average person. Much of the jargon (such as 'severely psychotic') was hugely offensive to service users. I waged battle to have the draft strategy translated into plain English and the more offensive terminology removed.

At first, this met with a little success, as some fellow members of the group were also anxious to make the final document more accessible. However, despite agreements made at meetings, subsequent revised documents still contained professional jargon.

Following surrender to semantic frustration, I tried to effect other change. I then sought to enforce the largely social model agenda outlined in the original need assessment, and also to have key user phrases inserted into the document, such as 'involvement at every level', 'user-run services' and 'user evaluation', etc. This met with some success, as Government guidelines at the time included such provision.

I did not take into account that all of the non-user representatives were major stakeholders in preserving the medical model (ultimately, their jobs and long-established links and friendships with hospital-based service providers being potentially affected).

In hindsight, I can now see that provision, such as community-run talking treatments (priorities in local need assessments), were always going to be at the bottom of the strategic purchasing charts. Tradition and 'the-devil-you-know' are always safe options and require, as a rule, less risk.

For instance, crisis services to be developed and run by the voluntary sector always headed the agenda, but seemed permanently in the planning stages and without resources. Strangely, resources were forthcoming when a local NHS trust had established a 'crisis service' and there were no competitors in the voluntary sector. Despite requests at every meeting for copies of the strategy budget to assist me in my 'participation', the only financial reports I ever received were historical. No budget access; no real involvement in decision making.

I accept that the lack of flexibility and creativity in designing the strategy was largely a result of rigid Government guidelines in policy formation, strict local deadlines and paid members' time management, all of which left little room for manoeuvre. There were no agreed user involvement guidelines and no related budget.

Taunts were also made about my 'representation'. Whom did I purport to represent? This argument would usually arise when I had touched a raw nerve, mostly after I had criticised the geographical or other practicalities of certain aspects of the strategy. I became sick and tired of reciting that I was the only democratically elected member, that I was also local, unpaid and the only ethnic minority representative serving on the group.

I would also occasionally remind the group that I, too, was very much in favour of better representation, particularly from the local Black community and from front-line staff, who could determine the practicalities of direct service provision outlined in the strategy. This was not followed up for one reason or another, probably because professional members working on the strategy seemed to be very over-worked and did not honestly have the time to recruit a more democratic membership.

As an Irish person, I encountered no direct racism from the strategy group. All of the members were well intentioned, very hardworking and committed to making a fine job of the strategy and its implementation. Attendance was always prompt and consistent.

But for me, culture is always difficult at such forums, especially when the dominant culture is professionalism and bureaucracy, regardless of the racial mix. My prior experience of psychiatry bred distinct power classifications between human beings in me, and it took time to get over my own perceived inferiority. Feelings and emotions are also generally alien to planning meeting proceedings. There is a huge pressure to conform to established manners and protocol; difficult if there is emotional attachment to the subject matter.

Many members of the group had problems adapting to my frequent method of communication by feeling, rather than by emotional detachment. Over a period of time, I had difficulty with this. There was a 'conform to protocol or be excluded' pressure. In order to participate more effectively, I seemingly had to withdraw my more explicit feelings in favour of a more logical approach. As someone who had discovered a few things about myself, I could see personal danger in this.

Part of my 'schizophrenia' was an absolute denial and repression of my own feelings in favour of a 'logical model' of being. I could see it was easier for the group if I changed, rather than disrupt the pervading culture and generate collective change. This was human, not malicious and I am guilty of having placed similar conforming pressures on others.

This personal dilemma was coupled with a realisation that there was little on the table to which I could claim real participation or ownership. The recommendations of the local need assessment were heavily diluted, absent or allocated to a traditional provider at this stage. I also felt that there was an unconscious strategy at work to keep me in a state of perpetual anger, thus conforming to the 'loud self-interested user' stereotype and resulting in my not having any marked effect on the strategy. I resigned from the group in late 1997.

Overall, my involvement in local strategic planning was not an empowering experience. It seemed I had been beating a drum on the sidelines of the main group for over a year. It seemed I irritated a lot of people with my noise, although I did get personal pleasure from my own rhythms. I achieved little, if anything, for local service users by my involvement. I had, however, met Government requirements for 'user involvement' at a strategic level.

I would not currently recommend involvement at a public sector strategic level to any service user.

Key points

⌘ After (mainly adverse) experiences of mental health services, the author became a member of the management committee of a MIND local association, where his 'input as an Irish person and a service user' was valued. Irish people are excluded from the management of organisations in the author's locality. However, these individuals are over-represented 'in ill health and disadvantage statistics'.

⌘ The author was invited to be a member of the local council's disability subcommittee, where he lobbied for mental health service user representation. The discriminatory remarks of a councillor went unchallenged.

⌘ As a member of a mental health strategy group, the author found a lack of black representation; maintenance of the *status quo* and of individuals' power; adherence to a medical model; and jargon 'offensive to service users'.

⌘ There was a lack of resources to implement plans. The author was denied financial information, so was unable to participate meaningfully in decision making. The group had no guidelines for service user participation.

⌘ Other members questioned the author's 'representativeness' as a service user, particularly when he criticised strategy. His suggestions to improve representativeness were not taken up, and he 'was the only democratically elected member'.

⌘ The author's experience of the mental health strategy group was disempowering. A specific protocol was imposed, and this did not allow for the expression of feelings.

given on how this is to be achieved. Participation where it does exist can be little more than lip service paid to the ideal, as the underlying ideology and decision-making structures have never really been tackled to date. There is a danger that participation may remain an elusive concept. Moreover, human services have an enormous capacity for destructiveness (Brandon, 1991). Providers set out with a set of principles and are diverted by a forest of hidden agendas, powerful vested interests and unconscious drives, all of which may lead to an ideological model of services becoming completely inconsistent with what users and staff actually experience and what they want and need (Brandon, 1991).

It must also be stressed that adequate resources are needed to back up consumer idealism. A changed culture is not likely to last long if there are not the resources to underpin the initiatives; if there is not enough money available then services are likely to be budget-led rather than user- or needs-led, shaped by financial constraints rather than by what people want or prefer. User-led services are not a cheap option. However, lack of money is no excuse for continuing to provide inappropriate or unacceptable services or for stopping users having their say in what happens (Croft and Beresford, 1993).

The following paragraph describes the philosophy behind the ideals of the drive towards consumerism in the health service.

Users should be involved in their own health care. Clients and carers should jointly agree individual care programmes and networks of support instead of people being channelled into the current limited services. Professionals need to work with clients rather than doing things to them or for them (Smith, 1998). They need to listen to clients and act on the knowledge gained rather than responding to diagnoses or labels (Hutcheson and Lucas, 1995). Participation is about working in partnership. It requires professionals to recognise the expertise and experience of the person who needs support in his or her daily life. This does not mean diminishing the expertise and experience of the practitioner, but rather putting this at the disposal of the clients. Participation is about sharing knowledge and experience, each to the other, in order to establish jointly what someone's needs are, and how they can best be met.

The experience of illness is largely characterised by loss of control over one's physical and/or mental state, one's environment and even one's freedom to make decisions on one's own behalf. If contact with professional care givers further limits people, or prevents them gaining control over their lives then it challenges the legitimacy of the service. Patients' and professionals' interrelationships are vital in promoting a sense of worth and competence. Practitioners should use their skills and experience to promote choice and control in clients' lives (Maxwell and Weaver, 1984). The last important point to make on partnership principles is that Rigge, in 1994, highlights the fact that in getting users to take more responsibility in healthcare service planning and delivery it is important to stress that partnership is in a health service rather than an illness service. Without success in this area, increasing consumer involvement will only lead to a downward spiral of clamouring demand being met with clinical refusal leading to dissatisfaction. Clients as partners in health care must be alert to the current political and managerial climate in NHS developments, understanding professionals' constraints as well as focusing on their own needs.

The elderly population in Britain

The first essential point to document concerns the age statistics in British society. The lengthening expectation of life and a changing age structure have produced a population with a rising proportion of people over sixty-five years old. The rise is dramatic. In 1991, the sixty-five and older age group represented 15% of the population, compared with 5% in 1901. Although the elderly percentage of the population has changed little since the late 1970s, the greatest change is in those within the age group who are living well into their seventies, eighties and even nineties. There is a rising proportion of the over seventy-fives and an even greater rise in those living to eighty-five and beyond. By 2001, 12% of the elderly will be in this very elderly bracket compared with 8% in 1983. The total number of people over eighty-five will rise by 54% between 1983 and 2003 (Abercrombie and Wade, 1988). These are the statistical facts and they carry with them a certain amount of presumed issues and problems for social services and health services. This is partly a question of the so-called 'burden of dependency', ie. these are a non-earning section of the population and they take up a disproportionate share of social security and health resources. For example, those aged sixty-five and over account for over a third of all NHS prescriptions and about 45% of acute hospital bed occupation. A substantial proportion of the elderly live alone. A third of the over sixty-fives do so, and the proportion increases with age. Many of these people will feel lonely and socially isolated especially if they are very old and relatively inactive.

Stereotypical views of the elderly

Western society values youth above all else. Ageism is alive and active in Britain today. Society generally holds negative stereotypes and attitudes about elderly people, and providers of health care are not immune to these. Stereotypical beliefs are cultural, reflecting political, economic and social relations. They are primarily reflections mirroring contemporary society, and shift as the structure of society shifts, but only slowly. Elderly people, as a group, are marginalised in a society which values youth and many suffer systematic exclusion from valued, contributing and participatory roles in the community. As with all stereotypes, the view assumes that all members of the group being described share the same characteristics. The negative stereotype of the elderly includes beliefs about dependency, frailty, ill health, poverty, physical and mental disabilities.

Although these facts and figures are true statistically, the elderly are not a homogenous group of people. If a third of the over sixty-fives live alone, two thirds of the same group do not live alone. Many are very active socially and have an active family life. Many are financially independent with a good quality of life and a high standard of living generally. Not only are many of the over sixty-fives independent, a large majority maintain good health and relative physical fitness with undiminishing mental capabilities. Far from requiring support from families, a great many are in fact vital to the stability of their families, actively giving support to children and grandchildren, sometimes practically, sometimes emotionally and often financially. But the demographic time bomb is ticking (Jackson, 2000). We are all living longer, healthier lives. By 2025, it is estimated that one third of the UK population will be over sixty and that is some size of a group to marginalise.

Elderly clients and the healthcare system

The elderly are regarded by society as a group that is low in the power stakes: an ill-conceived stereotype when applied to individuals. The power differentials are widened when elderly people become ill, and even further widened when they become cognitively as well as physically impaired. When these inequalities in power are taken into a healthcare system which has an already established power inequality between professionals and patients, the power differential is huge. It should be stated that this is a powerlessness which is compounded by the fact that it is often accepted by many of the elderly patients themselves. Elderly patients, especially the very elderly of eighty-five plus, may hold the same views of themselves as does society generally (of their powerless state) and may also acknowledge and defer to the powerfulness of the professionals. They may even resist well-intentioned attempts by professionals to establish partnership principles and to involve them in their own health care, actively preferring to hand over all responsibility to those whom they believe 'know best' (Brooker, 1994). It can be seen that empowerment and partnership as principles and philosophies can be very difficult issues to tackle when elderly people come into contact with health and social services.

Management of the health care of the elderly

As with **all** interactions between health professionals and clients, the key to empowerment and regaining choice and control in patients' lives is in the relationship between the professional and individual elderly patient. The role of the health professionals who work within the healthcare system cannot be underestimated (Morris, 1993). Kitwood (1992) is referring to elderly patients with dementia when he says:

> *Personal well-being is affected by the care practice... .*
> *People can be lifted through sensitive caring or pushed*
> *towards apathy and despair by neglect or put downs.*

Every person, whatever their disability or impairment, deserves to be treated as we ourselves would wish to be treated. Good care honours personhood. This is especially important when caring for elderly clients. The acknowledgement and respect for their individual unique histories, abilities, tastes, preferences, vulnerabilities, strengths and needs, supportive interpersonal relationships and individual reassurance is of incalculable importance to all patients, but particularly to the elderly who have become ill and whose physical and mental powers may be failing. The philosophy is not easy to put into practice. Healthcare professionals are not immune to cultural stereotypical beliefs about the elderly as a group in society. The willingness to acknowledge that there is a disproportionate allocation of power between elderly clients and professional carers and to address that discrepancy is the battle half won.

Elderly people with mental illness

Society may regard elderly people suffering from mental illnesses as one of the least powerful groups of people. One quarter of those over eighty-five develop dementia and between 10–16% develop clinical depression (Audit Commission, 2000). Both illnesses can affect a person's ability to take control over their own lives. Ageism may have its part to play in health service staffs' attitudes to the psychosocial needs of the elderly (Brooker, 1994). One of the most disabling barriers faced by people with dementia is the all too common assumption that it is impossible to communicate effectively with them (Goldsmith, 1996). Lack of communication with professionals can lead to patients feeling isolated, depressed and with a hopelessness associated with the diagnosis and a perceived denial of opportunities (Kitwood and Benson, 1995). Dementia is a term for a cluster of symptoms and signs of intellectual and cognitive function being disrupted, and individuals vary in the way that their conditions progress. The illness may have minimal manifestation, or vary through mild, moderate to severe. People with dementia are no more a homogenous group than those with other illnesses and should be treated as individuals with equal human rights to privacy, dignity, independence, choice, rights and fulfilment (Social Services Inspectorate [SSI], 1989).

The degree of sensitive caring management has been shown to have an effect on whether or not an individual remains fairly well-preserved or deteriorates through the stages of dementia that are commonly described (Kitwood and Bredin, 1992). Even when people have severe dementia with a high degree of speech impairment, non-verbal signals are often exceptionally candid and revealing, giving out many indications relating to the presence or absence of well-being, especially to those who know them well. Informal family carers may be especially skilled in reading these signals and understanding the idiosyncratic nature of the patients' language (Kitwood and Bredin, 1992). Mental health services intervene not just at the medical level but also at a social and psychological level and so partnership principles and the encouragement of independence take on an even greater importance.

Informal carers of elderly clients

Almost all publications about clients working in partnership with professional healthcare providers focus on the patient as the client and not the carer. The Trent, *Health Guide to User Empowerment in Mental Health Care*, refers to service users at all stages of the document. It stated that:

> *While carers may wish to speak for their relatives, it is important to remember that their needs and perceptions are different from the needs and perceptions of patients.*

When patients have dementia their carers' views in this instance may assume a greater significance than in other disease scenarios. Patient, carer and professionals may all be in partnership together. The patient obviously has to be the main focus of the care package. Carers who look after their relatives with dementia for twenty-four hours a day should be considered users of the service too. They are people whose detailed knowledge of their relatives is vital to producing practical care plans. They are also people whose well-being is vital to the continuing best management of the patients with dementia, in that they carry out much of the care which the professionals have planned. By working with carers it is possible for health professionals to build up a picture of patients' lives, to infer their needs more effectively, and to be able to assess their preferred options for their care and future management (Smith, 1988).

Twigg and Atkin (1994) spotlight the carer, his or her relationship to the cared for, and the impact on this relationship of policy and practice. They highlight the ambiguous position of carers and delineate four ways in which they may be regarded by professionals and agencies. These are; 'resources', 'co-workers', 'co-clients' and as 'superceded' carers. These varying roles carry different implications of how much support is offered and whose interests are judged to be paramount. All these roles have power differentials. Relationships with carers is also a fraught area when attempting to instigate partnership principles. Both professional and carer may feel vulnerable in the relationship. Both may feel that they have expertise in the management of patient care. Negotiation and trust are critical factors in the interactions between professionals and carers.

Issues in user feedback on health services for elderly people

The involvement of service users in the evaluation of services is seen as good practice by virtually every writer on quality in health care. User feedback on their views of the care delivered has to be collected and acted upon under the terms of reference of clinical governance. Satisfaction questionnaires remain the major consumer feedback tools.

The largest section of health service users are elderly people, for some of whom completion of satisfaction questionnaires may have specific problems. The current cohorts which make up the elderly population have been shown to be more passive and accepting of the standards of care given (Woodward and Wallston, 1987). More research into the older generation's expectations about health care, and what factors make it a positive or negative experience is required. High satisfaction, when expressed, could just be an artefact of low expectations.

Many elderly people with physical and or mental disabilities may be non-responders to questionnaires. Physically reading smallish print and completing the questions may be problematical. Those with cognitive impairments may misunderstand the questions or lack the concentration to complete forms. Often their information is ignored. Nevertheless, the views of the elderly as the largest group of users are very important. If their views are not heard the people who make value judgements about the factors which make up a good quality service will be younger more consumer-focused cohorts, and their opinions may not reflect the needs and wishes of older generations — the largest group of service users.

Structured interviews conducted by skilful interviewers are likely to provide more reliable feedback than questionnaire surveys. In this way, views can be heard from those who might otherwise be silent.

The way forward

Although it has been stated that much more is written about empowerment of clients and partnership principles than is actually practised, and that training and guidelines for staff have lagged behind the extolling of the philosophy, documents are being published which give more practical guidance on the management of services which promote independence for older people. The Carers Act of 1995, *Better Services for Vulnerable People* (DoH, 1997), *Partnership in Action* (DoH, 1998), *Forget Me Not* (Audit Commission, 2000) and the soon to be published *National Service Framework* (DoH, 2000) all set out new standards for the care of older people. All are designed to improve quality and decrease inequalities in the service. Hopefully, these will have an effect on the decision-making structures. Local NHS clinical governance initiatives will monitor that practice matches the standards set. Other quality initiatives in patient management are emerging as good practice, such as dementia care mapping (Kitwood and Benson, 1995), multi-professional, multi-agency care planning to address individual needs, patient held healthcare records and carer held records for patients with dementia. Primary care teams with integrated teams and professionals can have access to more flexible services. All these initiatives may guide individual practitioners towards best practice when caring for vulnerable clients. However, the key to empowerment of these clients lies in the individual relationship between client and professional carers. This cannot be over emphasised. The healthcare system is about recognising common humanity where individual practitioners deliver care which promotes a sense of worth and competence.

Key points

❧ Individuals are marginalised if they fail to conform, eg. by being old or disabled. This is reinforced by services that accord little power to older people, with decisions being made 'for', rather than 'with' them.

❧ Much has been written about participation and empowerment, but with little guidance on implementation. Service user/carer participation may be affected by other (conflicting) interests and inadequate resources.

❧ Participation includes involving service users in their health care; listening to, and working in partnership with them; and enabling their choice and control.

❧ The number of older people in the UK, especially those over seventy-five, is increasing. However, there is considerable ageism, with stereotypical beliefs and exclusion. It is often not recognised that many older people have relatively good health and quality of life, and provide support for their families.

❧ Power inequalities increase when elderly people are ill. This is reinforced by some health services, and some older people's internalisation of ageist attitudes.

❧ Key aspects of relevance to the care of elderly people include; valuing and respecting the individual, effective communication and enabling independence.

❧ Professionals should recognise the carers of elderly people as partners in care and as service users, with their own needs.

❧ More research is needed on older individuals' experiences of health care. Researchers should take these people's often low expectations into account. Methods should reflect their needs and any sensory and cognitive difficulties.

❧ Several central Government documents, local clinical governance initiatives and recent professional innovations provide impetus for increased empowerment and partnership with elderly people and their carers. Above all, professional-client relationships are 'the key to empowerment'.

References

Abercrombie N, Wade A (1988) *Contemporary British Society.* Polity Press, Cambridge

Audit Commission (2000) *Forget Me Not: Mental Health Services for Older People.* Audit Commission, London

Brandon D (1991) I*nnovation without change — consumer power in psychiatric services.* Macmillan Education Ltd, London

Brooker D (1994) Listening to the silent majority — issues in user feedback on health services for elderly people. *Br J Nurs* **6**(3): 159–62

Burgess AC, Burns J (1990) Partners in care. *Am J Nurs* **90**(6): 73–5

Croft S, Beresford P (1993) *Getting involved — a practical manual. Open services project.* Joseph Rowntree Foundation, BL catalogue record ISBN 0-9517554-1-2

Department of Health (1995) The Carers' Recognition and Service Act. DoH, London

Department of Health (1997) *Better Services for Vulnerable people,* EL (1997) 62, CI (97) 24.1997.

Department of Health (1998) *Partnerships in Action.* NHS Executive, London

Goldsmith M (1996) *Hearing the voices of people with dementia — opportunities and obstacles.* Jessica Kingsley Publishers, London

Hutcheson L, Lucas (1995) Mind Publication Mind SE.

Jackson A (2000) *The Book of Life. One man's search for the wisdom of age.* Indigo Press, London

Justice B, McBee G (1978) A client satisfaction survey as one element in evaluation. *Community Mental Health J* **14**: 248–52

Kitwood T (1991/2) *Evaluating quality care in formal settings.* ADS Newsletter 1991/2 Dec/Jan: 5

Kitwood T, Bredin K (1992) Towards a theory of dementia care: personhood and well-being. *Ageing Soc* **12**: 269–87

Kitwood T, Bredin K (1992) *Person to person: a guide to the care of those with failing mental powers.* 2nd edn. Gale Centre Publications, Essex

Kitwood T, Benson S, eds (1995) *The New Culture of Dementia Care.* Hawker Publications, London

Maxwell R, Weaver N (1984) Public participation in health: towards a clearer view. In: Smith H, *Collaboration for Change — Discussion paper, Partnership between service users, planners and managers of the NHS, 1988.* King's Fund Centre, London, No 871/140

Morris J (1997) Promoting choice and control. In: Reading P *Community Care and the Voluntary Sector.* Venture Press, Birmingham

Morris T (1993) Cost containment and the ethical foundations of the professional-client relationship: the case of physicians. *Prof Ethics* **2**(1–2): 89–111

Radke, Stam HJ, eds (1994) Foucault. In: *Power/Gender: Social relations in themes and practice.* Sage Publications, London

Rigge M (1994) Involving patients in clinical audit. *Qual Health Care* **3**(suppl): 2–5

Saunders P (1995) Encouraging patients to take part in their own care. *Nurs Times* **91**(9): 42–3

Smith H (1988) *Collaboration for Change — Discussion paper — Partnership between service users, planners and managers of the NHS.* King's Fund Centre, London, No. 871/140

Social Services Inspectorate (1989) *Homes are for Living In.* HMSO, London

Twigg J, Atkin K (1994) Carers perceived. Open University Press, Buckingham. In: Humphries B, ed (1996) *Critical Perspectives on Empowerment.* Venture Press, Birmingham

Webb A, Hobdell M (1980) Co-ordination and teamwork in the health and personal social services. In: Webb A, Lonsdale S, Briggs, Thomas L, eds. *Teamwork in Personal Social Services and Health Care: British and American perspectives.* Croome Helm, London.

Williams GH (1989) Hope for the humblest: The role of self help in chronic illness. *Sociology of Health and Illness* **11**(2): 135–57

Woodward NJ, Wallston BS (1987) Age and health care beliefs: Self-efficacy as a mediator of low desire for control. *Psychol Ageing* **2**: 3–8

10

Empowerment in mental health: the therapeutic community model

Anthony Bree, Penelope Campling, Susan Liderth

Penelope Campling (psychiatrist)

The practice of psychiatry has to be understood within the context of the society in which it exists. Because mental disorders directly affect behaviour, psychiatrists have legal powers invested in them. Unlike other doctors, our practice is always a precarious balance between protecting society and caring for an individual patient.

This chapter will focus on 'therapeutic communities' — a model of psychiatric practice which most obviously encompasses ideas of citizenship and empowerment. Therapeutic communities are deliberately structured in a way that encourages personal and collective responsibility and avoids unhelpful dependency on professionals. Patients are seen as bringing strength and creative energy into the therapeutic setting, and the peer group is seen as all important in establishing a strong therapeutic alliance. Patients (often referred to as residents) have a significant involvement in decision making and the practicalities of running the unit: this is understood to be part of the therapy and gives them an experience of their own potency.

Therapeutic community ideas have their roots in various religious and political movements and most obviously, develop some of the ideas espoused by Tuke and the Moral Treatment movement in the late eighteenth and early nineteenth century, for example, the importance of work, a healthy environment and warm relations (Kennard, 1998). Therapeutic communities, as we know them today, developed from two visionary innovations between 1942 and 1948, known as the Northfield experiments (Harrison, 2000).

Army psychiatric services were faced with hundreds of psychologically traumatised soldiers and the expectation that they were to help as many as possible recover to a state where they could return to the front line. The psychiatrists at Northfield Hospital decided to focus on the unit as a whole, rather than on individuals and structured the wards as communities, encouraging mutual support and co-operation (in some ways similar to life in the army) with group discussions to examine and understand the process. They saw the whole community as both the patient and the instrument of treatment and the aim was the education and training of the community in the problems of neurotic defences and interpersonal relationships (Harrison, 2000). This idea was later known as the 'living-learning' experience (Jones, 1968).

At the same time, Maxwell Jones was developing a unit along similar lines at Mill Hill, helping soldiers suffering from what was known as 'effort syndrome'. Lectures about the physiological basis of their symptoms gradually led to more open discussions, more experienced patients giving information to newer patients, and a less rigid demarcation between doctors, nurses and patients. Maxwell Jones went on to become the director of a new unit set up to tackle the problems of 'unemployed drifters' at Belmont Hospital in Surrey. Belmont was renamed Henderson Hospital in 1958 and is perhaps, the best known therapeutic community of its kind (Jones, 1979).

During the nineteen sixties and seventies, a number of democratic therapeutic communities were set up in different parts of the country, sharing some basic ideological principles but evolving in individual ways according to local needs and resources. The eighties and nineties saw many of these units close — perhaps because they were antithetical to the prevailing philosophy within society, particularly the promotion of individualism at the expense of collectivism (Kennard, 1998). It seems that the tide is changing again and the last few years have seen the opening of new therapeutic communities within the NHS, with others in the planning stage and a parallel expansion within the prison service and voluntary sector.

Although therapeutic community practice overlaps with other services, the structured attempt to raise the status of patients and the all embracing 'culture of enquiry', mean that therapeutic communities have a cohesive philosophy, despite some variations in detail between particular communities. By definition, therapeutic communities are continually evolving. This makes them difficult to categorise, define and study. One of the lessons learnt over the last fifty years, is that, whatever the set-up, institutionalisation will occur unless the 'culture of enquiry' is such as to question the *status quo* on an ongoing daily basis (Hinshelwood, 2001).

Rapaport and a team of sociologists were invited to study Henderson Hospital and wrote a book, *Community as Doctor* (Rapaport, 1960). Four principles emerged which are often quoted as defining the work of a therapeutic community: democracy, reality confrontation, permissiveness and communalism. These should not be seen as absolutes but rather as principles in tension with each other. For example, the reality of professional accountability cannot be ignored and while it is vital that all community members have a significant voice in decisions that affect their lives, it is important to be realistic and clear about the limits of democratic decision making and the responsibility of professionals to provide a 'safe frame' for therapeutic work. Likewise, permissiveness would usually be limited to the verbal expression of feelings and strongly confronted if it led to other members of the community being hurt, damaged or feeling excluded. Racist comments, for example, would not be allowed to go unchallenged in modern therapeutic communities.

In addition to the small cohesive units sometimes referred to as 'therapeutic communities proper', or democratic analytic therapeutic communities (Clark, 1999; Kennard, 1998), an important part of the development of therapeutic community practice has involved work with people with mental illness.

This was:

> ... described as the 'therapeutic community approach'... from the 1950s until the 1970s was what many psychiatrists meant by the phrase 'social psychiatry'. A World Health Organization report (WHO, 1953) [commented that]... 'The most important single factor in the efficacy of the treatment given in a mental hospital appears... to be an intangible element which can only be described as its atmosphere'... . Too many psychiatric hospitals give the impression of being an uneasy compromise between a general hospital and a prison. Whereas, in fact, the role they have to play is different from either, it is that of the therapeutic community.
>
> ... The fundamental premise of social therapy was that for people spending a long time [in hospital]... the way that they lived, the work they did, their personal relationships, the regime with its rewards and punishments, were more important for their... rehabilitation than the medical treatment they might receive...

(Clark, 1999, p. 32, quoting WHO, 1953, pp. 17–18)

Although there have been many changes in the intervening years, most noticeably the improvement in psycho-pharmacological approaches and the move from hospital to community management of patients, the therapeutic community approach continues to raise fundamental questions about the nature and management of mental health problems.

The application of therapeutic community ideas has had a significant impact on the practice of psychiatry in the past. The need for the caring asylum has not gone away, and, with many acute admission wards in therapeutic crisis, is becoming a pressing problem once again (McGeorge and Lindow, 2000). The task is to provide therapeutic social environments where people are 'able to express feelings and views, engage in fulfilling activity and participate in decisions affecting their lives' (Byrt, 1999, p. 73).

Therapeutic community ideas continue to raise fundamental questions and challenge us all to think more positively and creatively about the potential within our patients.

Susan Liderth (resident)

When I arrived at the therapeutic community from an acute ward, I was surprised at the amount of freedom I could enjoy. Some new residents ask for permission to go out and how long they can stay out. We are free to come and go as we please, outside of the timetable of meetings and other activities. As residents, we play a part in setting rules and boundaries. We often test them and sometimes alter them. The culture of the place changes with the coming and going of residents. For example, we organise work rotas and will challenge each other if jobs aren't done. The way we do the jobs changes according to each person's methods and how they pass on instructions to a new resident.

As we progress through the 'Lodge', our confidence grows. An obvious example of this is chairing meetings. (We chair all community meetings: two a-day, every morning and evening — I see them as the backbone of the community.)

'I'll never chair a meeting!' I've heard this comment so many times, yet every resident takes a turn to chair meetings for a month. After chairing meetings in the Lodge, one resident went on to chair a meeting outside the 'Lodge' to sort out her housing needs.

We also sponsor new residents, look after them in their first few days. During my early months at the Lodge, I thought, 'I'll never be able to sponsor a new resident', yet I did, and it wasn't as bad as I expected. Everybody takes their turn, these roles are not what most of us expected and we grow in ways that we don't expect. We support each other, so even the most daunting job isn't tackled alone. This is something else I've gained by participating in the life of the Lodge: the value of receiving and giving support.

It is not just about therapy but learning life skills, taking control of our lives, having a say in our treatment. This feels more powerful and relevant than listening passively to 'experts' telling me what to do. They often do more harm than good. We work with the 'Lodge' staff, we challenge and support them. They do the same with us.

Before we join the Lodge, most of us on medication make a commitment to reduce and eventually come off it. We decide, with encouragement, when to reduce and when to stop. This type of empowerment can lead to conflict when some residents resist reducing their 'meds'. But eventually, nearly everybody decides to stop taking them.

I have had rules unfairly imposed on me in the past, so I often kicked against rules while I was at the Lodge. I wanted to test them, also to see how safe I was within their framework. The rules can be changed, but only after discussion with the whole community. For example, if a resident has persistently broken a rule, we can vote for them to take five days' leave to think about their future at the Lodge. We can also vote to advise the consultant that a resident should leave, but this rarely happens. Some of us kick against boundaries to avoid looking at painful issues. We point this out to each other, often more bluntly than staff. We become able to recognise parts of ourselves by seeing them in other residents. We identify with each other and feel less alone. Sometimes, I've felt like my own therapist by listening to and watching other residents.

The community needs to be strong and safe, for bullying does go on and empowerment becomes abuse. Staff are not aware of what happens and bullying comes to light when the bully leaves. This has happened at the Lodge and there is always the potential for this without strong members of the community to challenge abusive residents.

Participating in a healthy way within a healthy community is a new experience for most of us. Seeing it work, seeing longer-staying residents give insightful feedback to each other in community meetings and psychotherapy groups, gave me some faith in the Lodge. I saw people taking control over their lives, giving up their trails of self-destruction, replacing them with healthier ways of coping, finding ways for themselves. I have learnt to take control so my impulses don't control me: to direct my feelings outwards, to stop punishing myself.

Sometimes it feels as if staff play lip service to the idea of community, when decisions are made without discussion, like granting five days' leave without consulting the community. This feels disempowering. On the other hand, I've felt safer and very relieved when staff tell residents to leave when drugs have been taken. The framework gives way at times but this reflects life. We talk about it, hopefully learn from it, and move on.

I've gained self-respect by giving feedback in meetings and groups. It's enriching when staff and residents listen to me and when they give me feedback. It makes me feel alive, useful, part of something positive. I've learnt to listen to others' opinions, to allow them room to express themselves and participate more equally. The community has been strong enough to challenge the more outspoken and omnipotent — making residents appear in a way that is not totally crushing. It enables us to learn to express ourselves in ways less damaging to others.

We decide when to become a day resident, when to join 'Next Step' and when to leave. This made me feel in control and I did not feel as if I was being kicked out.

By participating at the Lodge, I've felt empowered, I've learnt to control my self-destructive impulses, to take control of my life. After leaving, feelings still verge out of control territory, but the helter-skelter crazy path of chaos becomes boringly more ordered and slowly more bearable. On leaving the Lodge, I find life is much the same but I have changed and struggle to readjust and refit into society: trying to accept that I can participate as a more rounded person. Frightening and disorienting, with time it comes. I have a right to say how someone's behaviour or words make me feel. I take control by verbalising my feelings, I don't direct them inwards with the venom of the past.

There are still times I want to cut and get drunk, to act out, but I can't. I have tried, but I have changed more deeply than I realise, more than I want. I have to deal with my feelings in new ways. I bear them, live with them and they have not destroyed me — yet.

Anthony Bree (mental health nurse)

In the following section, I explain how we try to empower patients in a therapeutic community setting. We find it helpful to think of empowerment as a developmental process which requires a working-through of psychological and emotional conflicts around power and dependence in order to bring about **internal** change, within both systems and individuals. Change inevitably involves exposure to risk and uncertainty; attitudes which are invested with both emotional and psychological security may be called into question and need to be reformulated or rejected altogether. The therapeutic community principles recognise the inter-relationship between personal problems and social context; work is directed at influencing both.

Francis Dixon Lodge is one of the few residential democratic-analytic therapeutic communities which remain from the heyday of the therapeutic community movement in the 1960s. What originated as a conventional psychiatric ward, has evolved into a social organisation which aspires to open communication and democracy. Large and small groups are used to talk about personal problems. Psychotherapy and sociotherapy enable staff and residents to work collaboratively to explore the day-to-day business of relating and living together. The term 'sociotherapy', or more precisely social therapy, has been defined as:

> *... an attempt to help people to change by affecting the way in which they live. It is based on the observation that people are shaped by the way they live, unfortunately often for the worse.*

(Clark, 1974)

We try to maintain the principle of a 'culture of enquiry' (Main, 1983); there is an understanding that everyone and every event may be subjected to scrutiny in order to provide a learning and empowering experience. Everyone is regarded as having something of value to contribute, whatever their background.

According to Haigh (1999), there are five essential ingredients of therapeutic culture:

- attachment: a culture of belonging
- containment: a culture of safety
- communication: a culture of openness
- involvement: a culture of participation and citizenship
- agency: a culture of empowerment.

The overall aim of the therapeutic community is to raise the status of residents so that they assume responsibility and control of their own lives, rather than being dependent upon medical and nursing care. It is not always a comfortable place in which to work; the expectation of openness applies equally to staff and we are rightly expected to account for ourselves honestly when challenged, rather than take refuge behind a professional façade.

In the following examples, I briefly describe three aspects of community life which present both empowerment opportunities and dilemmas for its members.

The assessment interview

The decision to admit a new resident to the unit, like other agreements in therapeutic community life, is the outcome of a collaborative process. After an initial meeting with staff, an interview is arranged with a panel, consisting of two staff members and three residents. The individual will be invited to 'take the floor' and explain to the panel what aspects of life they are unhappy with and how the community might be able to help. Each person has the right to vote for or against admission; the composition of the panel means that collectively, residents can override the decision of staff.

Most psychiatric patients have extensive experience of being interviewed by professional mental health workers. An implicit assumption of the medical model is that the interviewer, with the benefit of professional training and clinical experience, will try to arrive at an objective understanding of the patient's presenting and potential problems in order to identify the 'solution'. Unfortunately, the patient's need to understand himself or herself can easily get overlooked. Unless patients can 'own' solutions as emanating from within their own creativity and resources, promoting autonomy and boosting self-esteem, we risk reinforcing a passive dependency, where unacknowledged hostility is acted out through repeated failure to achieve therapeutic aims.

There is, nevertheless, an element of clinical objectivity in therapeutic community work; one of the most important tasks is to try and anticipate what difficulties might arise so that we do not set applicants up to fail.

Residents can make an important contribution to the selection process because their capacity to empathise with the person seeking help is largely based on identification through personal experience. Empathic understanding and advice communicated from such a position can be enormously influential because of its authenticity. At the same time, however, it presents a dilemma for residents: on the one hand, there is a powerful desire to accept the applicant which is driven by identification with the individual's despair and problems; on the other, there is a conflicting need to protect oneself and the community from the pain of adjustment, just like any family having to accommodate a new arrival. These factors must be weighed along with an assessment of the applicant's motivation to change, a willingness to take responsibility for their behaviour and the capacity of the community to contain disturbance. The predicament appeals to the adult part of the personality and promotes psychological growth if managed constructively.

Ownership of community rules

Many residents who seek help from a therapeutic community have grown up in families where parental discipline has either been absent entirely or rigid, arbitrary and punitive. Those with histories of abuse have had their developing personal boundaries intruded upon at such a vulnerable age that the consequences can be catastrophic for the individual concerned and those who get close to them; in very simple terms, little emotional demarcation exists between self and other. The capacity to contain intense feeling is often limited and may find expression through anti-social behaviour, which in turn, elicits an equally negative response from the parent or an alternative authority figure. Sanctions of increasing severity have to be resorted to as the growing child becomes more powerful, reinforcing in his or her mind a belief that the world is an uncaring place where rules exist only to maintain dominance of the strong over the weak.

One way of changing this script is reflected in the therapeutic community principle of 'democracy'. This means that each member of the community has the right to question or express an opinion about any aspect of community life and, if necessary, vote for things to be done differently. This includes many of the rules. While some are not negotiable, for example, the principle that violence against anyone will not be tolerated, much community meeting time is spent negotiating boundaries and discussing infringements. An important example at Francis Dixon Lodge is the rule which until recently, forbade residents to consume alcohol off the premises during the Monday to Friday therapy programme. There were many good reasons for retaining such a rule, but unless agreement on its usefulness could be reached by a consensus of community members, enforcement of the boundary usually fell on the staff, which inevitably set up an unreflective, persecutory 'us-and-them' split, undermining the 'therapeutic alliance': the notion that staff and residents work collaboratively for the overall good of the residents. The residents decided, following a vote, to allow themselves the privilege of going to the pub in the evening for a 'social drink'. This change required residents to shoulder extra responsibility for one another, and think through situations more objectively as a price of additional freedom. Who would make the distinction between a 'social drink' and intoxication? Who would determine the consequences if somebody overstepped the limit? How would residents with a history of alcohol abuse be affected by the change? Should they be invited along too and expected to abstain or left behind to watch TV? The inter-relatedness of empowerment, participation, personal and collective responsibility might be regarded as strands of an invisible thread from which the very fabric of the therapeutic community is woven.

Creative aspects of crisis

Many people might argue that stability is preferable to crisis, which upsets the state of homeostatic equilibrium that living organisms and social systems strive to maintain. While true integration results in true stability, a delusion of stability may be created by the expulsion of a feeling, idea, person or group which is perceived by the organism or system as a threat (Yalom, 1995). Ronald Higgins describes the human factor as the greatest potential source of global crisis: political inertia, or the profound failure of governments to face up to the true global agenda goes unchallenged because they provide convenient containers for the collective projection of our own indifference and preoccupation with our own selfish priorities (Higgins, 1978).

For centuries, societies have preserved a sense of psychological stability by splitting off collective disturbance and projecting it into seriously disturbed individuals or groups who were either persecuted or incarcerated. Crisis, on the other hand, can be re-framed, and be regarded as a step towards wholeness, although a potentially uncomfortable step, depending on the degree of adjustment required. The real crisis of care in the community is whether society is prepared to acknowledge, own and integrate the darker, disturbed aspects of human nature which, in reality, belong to us all. 'Disability is superimposed by the rejection mechanisms stemming from cultural attitudes' (Hunt, 1959). In the 'blame culture' we have imported from North America over the last two decades, driven by litigation, individualism and an obsession with service economies, there is a risk that a balanced attitude to crisis will become endangered. If psychiatry is expected to anticipate and deal with crisis by the most repressive and cheapest means possible, rather than allow, contain and work with it while resolution occurs, then it is hard to see how ideas such as empowerment and participation can ever be more than tokenism. We regard crisis as an indication that long-established, but frequently immature and self-defeating coping mechanisms, are beginning to fail in protecting an individual or even the community group from anxiety.

If the situation is contained, the nature of the anxiety and underlying feelings can be explored, tolerated and survived. A resident can call a crisis meeting at any hour of the day or night, drawing on the experience, support and containment of the whole community. A fundamental principle of this approach is the idea that we are all a combination of strength and vulnerability, wisdom and ignorance, sickness and health, whether staff member or resident. While residents are protected from the final responsibility for crisis management decisions, their counsel and involvement is always sought. Thus, both risk and scope for creative intervention are more widely spread than would normally be the case.

Everyone is potentially open to learning in crisis situations. Mary came to the Lodge with a history of terrible childhood abuse, which had taken place in her bedroom. In response to 'flashbacks' she would disappear to her room and sometimes cut herself. When other community members, concerned about her safety, knocked on her door, she would not respond, so that finally, they had to enter her room uninvited. Eventually, Mary learned to trust and ask for help and support when she was distressed. The cutting gradually stopped. Several months later, a new resident was admitted who also retreated to her room and refused to open the door when in crisis. This time, Mary was one of the 'helpers' who went into the new resident's room uninvited.

In the community meeting the following morning, Mary reflected on how awful she had felt at being put in the position of having to intrude into the privacy of someone else's room. It was not until that moment, that she realised how others must have felt when she had acted out a similar situation.

This is the **real** nature of empowerment which can be learned through participation.

Experiencing how one is experienced by others involves a shift in responsibility to the individual as insight develops. With insight and responsibility, choices open up where previously they were limited.

> **Key points**
>
> ⌘ Therapeutic communities empower residents through opportunities to participate in decision making and responsibility and express feelings and views. 'Unhelpful dependency on staff' is avoided, and residents are enabled to contribute 'strength and creative energy'. Staff maintain professional accountability.
>
> ⌘ These organisations originate in the moral treatment movement of the late eighteenth and early nineteenth centuries, and in innovations in military hospitals in World War II. Therapeutic communities flourished in the nineteen sixties and seventies, and their principles were applied in rehabilitation and other settings. Following the closure of many units, there has been a recent revival, with the opening of new therapeutic communities.
>
> ⌘ A former resident of a therapeutic community (Francis Dixon Lodge) found her stay empowering. She describes the amount of freedom, and the involvement of residents in 'setting rules and boundaries'. Residents gain confidence, support each other, learn life skills, have a say in their treatment, and gain control of their lives.
>
> ⌘ The breaking of rules and testing of boundaries are discussed so that people can understand themselves better. When bullying occurs, 'empowerment becomes abuse'.
>
> ⌘ Sometimes, staff make decisions without consulting residents, but at times, this can engender feelings of safety and relief. The therapeutic community enables self-respect and learning to 'listen to others' opinions'. Residents take control of their lives, decide when to leave, and develop positive ways of coping and dealing with feelings.
>
> ⌘ Staff at Francis Dixon Lodge see empowerment as a 'developmental process', involving the working through of conflicts to enable change. This is achieved through the exploration of life and relationships in the therapeutic community.

⌘ Efforts are made to maintain 'a culture of enquiry'. Every event in the life of the therapeutic community can 'provide a learning and empowering experience'. A therapeutic culture is engendered, characterised by belonging, safety, openness, involvement and empowerment.

⌘ 'Empowerment opportunities and dilemmas' are described in relation to assessment interviews of prospective residents, ownership of the rules of the community, and creative aspects of crisis.

⌘ As part of a 'blame culture', there are expectations in some health services that crises should be dealt with 'by the most repressive and cheapest means'. In contrast, in Francis Dixon Lodge, crises are used as opportunities for learning. An example is given to illustrate 'the real nature of empowerment which can be learned through participation'.

References

Byrt R (1999) Nursing: the importance of the psychosocial environment. In: Campling P, Haigh R, eds. *Therapeutic Communities: Past, Present and Future.* Jessica Kingsley Publishers, London: 63–75

Clark DH (1999) Social Psychiatry: The therapeutic approach. In: Campling P, Haigh R, eds. *Therapeutic Communities: Past, Present and Future.* Jessica Kingsley Publishers, London

Haigh R (1999) The quintessence of a therapeutic environment; five universal qualities. In: Campling P, Haigh R, eds. *Therapeutic Communities: Past, Present and Future.* Jessica Kingsley Publishers, London

Harrison J (2000) *Bion, Rickman, Foulkes and the Northfield Experiments.* Jessica Kingsley Publishers, London

Higgins R (1978) *The Seventh Enemy: The human factor in the global crisis.* Hodder and Stoughton, London

Higgins R (1980) The therapeutic community and the global crisis. *Int J Therapeutic Communities* **1**(1): 59–63

Hinshelwood RD (2001) *Thinking about Institutions. Milieux and madness.* Jessica Kingsley, London

Hunt RC (1959) Ingredients of a therapeutic programme. In: Caplan G (1959) *An Approach to Community Mental Health.* Tavistock, London

Jones M (1968) *Social Psychology in Practice: The idea of the therapeutic community.* Penguin, Harmondsworth

Jones M (1979) The therapeutic community, social learning and social change. In: Hinchelwood RD, Manning NP, eds. *Therapeutic Communities, Reflections and Progress.* Routledge and Kegan Paul Ltd, London

Kennard D (1998) *An Introduction to Therapeutic Communities.* Routledge, London

McGeorge M, Lindow V (2000) Safe in our Hands? *Mental Health Practice* **4**(4): 4– 6

Main TF (1983) The concept of the therapeutic community: variations and vicissitudes. In: Pines M, ed. *The Evolution of Group Analysis.* Routledge and Kegan Paul Ltd, London

Rapaport RN, Rapaport R, Rosow I (1960) *Community as Doctor.* Tavistock, London

World Health Organization (1953) *Expert Committee on Mental Health: 3rd Report.* WHO, Geneva

Yalom ID (1995) *The Theory and Practice of Group Psychotherapy.* 4th edn. Basic Books, New York

11

Women's needs in a medium secure unit: a former patient's perspective

Wendy Ifill

In my opinion, women are still treated as second-class citizens in many walks of life and this is no exception in the hospital environment. At the moment, I am detained in a medium secure unit, where I am one of only five women in a total of over fifty patients. This, in itself, puts the women in the unit in the minority and so could lead to their being left out. Female patients in a predominately male setting do not always receive services geared to their needs.

How has this been addressed in the unit I am in? Well, the first thing that happened was the establishment of the women's services group, of which I was a member. This was set up to look at women's needs in Arnold Lodge. The group developed a number of initiatives aimed at the women in the unit.

In a paper published prior to the setting up of the group, I described a mainly negative situation, where women were not getting much quality time (Ifill, 1998). However, in a later article, I was able to represent a much different picture, with access to women only groups (Ifill, 2002).

Many women in secure institutions lack self-esteem. This can manifest itself in different ways, but it can be harder to deal with in male company. Some females, due to their past histories, may have problems interacting with males. This can be for many reasons, but the number of women in hospital I have shared stories concerning physical, mental and sexual abuse at the hands of men, would indicate that such abuse is common.

I would like to urge women-only wards in secure environments. This would enable women to develop, have privacy and retain some manner of dignity. It would mean that they could live, while receiving treatment, in an atmosphere free of men, bearing in mind that often men have been the perpetrators of crimes against them. However, some women may choose to live in mixed sex environments.

I have been in a medium secure hospital for four years now and in that time, women have experienced many changes. Previously, the need for women to have their own space, although recognised, was not acted upon. About two years into my stay, an all-woman social group was set up, but this didn't succeed. I feel the reasons for this included the lack of structure: the groups were a bit hit and miss. Also, there was emphasis on the fact that because we were all women, we would naturally get on well together. In the autumn of 1998, some new groups were set up, solely for the women. These were activity based and seemed to work better than the chatty social group. They were mainly run by outside facilitators and ran at an agreed upon time each week.

'Women only' was the rule of the day and for me, it meant a great deal: a group in which I was not in competition with the men. However, of equal importance, I got the chance to work with the other women in the group.

People assume that women thrown together in a male environment, or even in a group on their own, will naturally get on. This was far from the truth in the ward setting, there was rivalry and competition between the women that often drove them poles apart. However, this competition did not seem so apparent in the activity groups set up for women. In addition to the Well Woman Clinic and input from WISH (Women in Secure Hospitals), the women's sessions that took place included Rhythms (music group), aerobics, relaxation, gym and aromatherapy. These groups were not set up as a means of segregating the men from the women, but to give the very few women in the unit some space. The groups, although not individual (apart from aromatherapy), bore the individual in mind. This was highlighted by the fact that the groups still went ahead, even if only one person attended.

A lot of the groups which ran were about learning new skills. This included Rhythms, a music group which initially began with percussion, drums and sax. It was not about becoming the world's next best drummer or saxophone player, it was about enjoyment, working as a team, boosting your self-confidence and learning new skills. The skills learnt in these groups were not just about becoming adept at the steps in aerobics or mastering the techniques of relaxation, they were about listening to what was going on around you, listening to what others have to say, following instructions, working together as a team to create a sound, or play a team game such as badminton or short tennis in the gym. In aromatherapy, each person was given a half an hour session. These sessions gave not only a chance to be pampered (although this was an added bonus), it was about trust in the aromatherapist, learning how to relax, learning about yourself and your body, having individual space and gaining confidence in yourself.

I thought that with the setting up of these new groups, there would be rumblings from the male population of the unit. On the whole, this was not the case, they seemed to accept the situation as it was.

Everybody needs to be given the element of choice, as well as to be allowed to be in control of their own destiny. Many women coming into secure units have not had the chance to do this. Their self-worth is often low and it is men who have taken away their self-respect, so you can imagine how they feel in a predominately male unit. Many women who find themselves in mental health services have often been there for some time and may lack self-esteem. They often find it difficult to express their distress, many use self-harm as a means of communicating stress or degrading themselves.

Women-only groups are not the complete answer to helping women but they may help in bridging the gap, and having been a participant of the groups, I feel that, along with other forms of treatment, they may help women to gain some confidence and self-respect, enabling them to move on.

There is lots to learn about the treatment of women in secure and medium secure hospitals. But, initiatives such as the one described here have got to be steps in the right direction.

Key points

- Women are treated as 'second class citizens', in wider society and in hospitals.

- Female patients in mixed gender medium secure units 'do not always receive services geared to their needs' because of the large majority of male patients.

- Many female patients have been abused by men. Women-only secure wards would enable their development, privacy and dignity.

- A women's services group, with the author as a member, was set up in the unit where she was a patient. The group developed initiatives in response to women's needs.

- A women's social group had been unsuccessful. However, following the establishment of the women's services group, women-only activity groups, mainly with external facilitators, were provided. These gave women space, reduced rivalry; and enabled the development of trust and acquisition of new skills.

- Women-only groups in secure units may also increase confidence and self-respect for individuals who are distressed, with limited self-esteem, and a lack of past opportunities for choice or control.

Reference

Ifill C (1998) One of a kind. *Nurs Times* **94**(27): 14–15
Ifill W (2002) Mad or just bad. *Mental Health Practice* **6**(3)

12

Participation and empowerment of users and carers in mental health services

Jenny Fisher

I write from the perspective of a carer and my experience of my son's illness and of supporting other carers and users of mental health services. I have worked as a volunteer with the national schizophrenia fellowship (NSF, now Rethink) and currently have the honour to be the national chairman. In addition, I am a member of Leicestershire community health council (CHC). My work with the CHC provides a balance between my continuing passionate interest in the treatment and care of people with severe mental illness and appreciation of the needs of individuals requiring care in other areas, such as learning disabilities and child and adolescent mental health. As a CHC member, I have gained an understanding of ways in which these fields compete with the acute services such as those for coronary heart disease and accident and emergency.

In this chapter, I am concerned with the empowerment and participation in health care of severely mentally ill people and their carers.

Individual rights to freedom and the Mental Health Act, 1983

Power is something which is shared in our society, and individuals have rights to make decisions for themselves and to live as they please within the law. These rights are recognised and respected by society, but when individuals develop severe mental illness, they may have these rights removed. Under the Mental Health Act 1983, power is given to the authorities to detain and take control of the individual's life, until (s)he is judged to have regained the capacity to do so.

There are clear guidelines to be followed when making the decision to detain, and safety clauses to ensure that the section is regularly reviewed and that the individual is not detained inappropriately. The Mental Health Act allows for the detention of individuals who have a severe mental disability, who are a danger to themselves or others, or who have a deteriorating illness.

Detention for deterioration has not been recognised recently and patients have been left at home to get steadily worse until crisis or danger is imminent. People with a severe mental illness have impaired cognitive function and may lose the capacity to make even small decisions.

When it becomes necessary to detain an individual, the aim must always be to get his or her co-operation as far as possible, without pressure: it may take longer but it will make the treatment more acceptable to the individual. Empowering the individual afterwards is about recovery and rehabilitation, returning to independence and resuming rights. Sectioning is clearly disempowering for the individual, but carers may welcome it as an opportunity to rest and for treatment to start. I see the purpose of the Mental Health Act as providing safety and sanctuary to ill people, but this has also been abused in recent times.

Diagnosis and labelling

There is a great deal talked about diagnoses, whether or not we should label people and whether labelling is disempowering. Perhaps it depends on the degree of disability. The diagnosis causes difficulties with getting a mortgage or life insurance, in job interviews and other areas. It is also true that without a diagnosis, it is difficult to penetrate the barriers to information and benefits. Perhaps, more importantly, it is the symptoms which need to be identified and treated early.

Our son's admissions to hospital have all been voluntary. When he was diagnosed with schizophrenia, two things happened: it enabled us to discover the national schizophrenia fellowship and get hold of information and support which empowered us, but it marked our son as a mentally ill person, disempowering him. However, it gave him the answer which he needed to know, explaining why he was unable to do what others do. He did not like it and said that for a long time he would wake, thinking perhaps it was all a dream.

Stigma and exclusion

Severe mental illness is stigmatising to all involved, the patients, staff and families, who may well feel isolated in the 'community'.

Users and carers come from the general public with its inhibitions and prejudices. Much of their belief comes from the media representations of mental illness. The effects of these devastating illnesses and its stigma reach beyond the individual's immediate family to the wider family and its social support networks, friends, work and leisure. Commonly, families are shunned, ostracised and disempowered .

A new report by the Mental Health Foundation, *Pull Yourself Together*, reveals that users feel that they are also discriminated against by their families (Mental Health Foundation, 2000). I think that this is true and I am always distressed to see the catastrophic loss of self-respect, the terrible guilt and the shame users and carers feel, and their ignorance about severe mental illness. I have read that many people who suffer a psychotic illness develop a post traumatic shock response, which I can well understand.

Severely mentally ill people can become extremely powerful and very threatening.

This may happen where a user lives with aged parents. I have spoken to elderly parents who have whispered into the telephone, fearful that their paranoid grown child will hear. Where the knot between parent and grown child is allowed to become too tight, it may not be possible to undo and can be dangerous, disempowering the carer.

Control

It may be that the user is behaving irrationally and needs to be controlled, especially if he or she is in a public place. The public's views of mental illness, already distorted by the media, may escalate the situation. On the other hand, the person's illness may be invisible, although his thinking is deeply impaired. It may also fluctuate. An eminent psychiatrist told me that for some people, the illness is a 'now you see it, now you don't' thing. Many family carers describe their visit to the general practitioner, where the patient is rational and collected, only to trash the house when they get home. The situation is seldom quite clear and this is wearing and distressing for all concerned. Where professionals have to control an individual, there are parallels with parents controlling their children.

Parents have to find ways of doing this without making the child feel insecure or unloved. Controlling the detained patient requires staff to act, while retaining respect for the individual's dignity. The situation is further complicated if there is aggression and a staff member or patient gets hurt. An aggressive act will be recorded and the patient labelled as aggressive which is disempowering. A wise and charming gentleman with schizophrenia once told me that as a psychiatric patient, you could never lose your temper. He was spot on.

Our son became very primitive in his behaviours when ill, especially in relation to self-care and table manners. Sometimes, people become difficult to like and this can be hard for professionals too. It is not an easy field of work. In situations where the professional has to provide care and control, (s)he needs to be well supported, especially when administering medication against the wishes of the individual. This also applies to the practice of restraint. Staff need good initial training and regular updating. Bungled restraint attempts are unhelpful to all concerned. In my view, psychiatric nurses are breaching their code of conduct if they have not acquired the skills needed for their job.

All of us are affected by opposing views in society about giving treatment or restraining without consent. This conflict of opinion provides a safeguard against malpractice and is empowering for the individual. But, I have anxieties about some of the tools used to gain control over vulnerable people. These include the police using CS gas and handcuffs and hospital staff's use of medication to induce sedation. Such measures must be used only as a last resort and after real consideration. In practice, they will make a frightened patient more frightened and add to the task of restoring confidence and co-operation later. Patients have remarkably clear memories about the treatment they have received.

Disabilities

Users spend a great deal of time thinking about how they came to be ill, how it is that they cannot do the things that others do, like getting up in the morning, working, being able to cope with what other people cope with, further lowering their already low self-esteem. They need to know that they are not just lazy and feckless but have a severe illness which disables them, and they also need to know they can improve.

By the time we knew our son's diagnosis, we had been in deep trouble for two years.

He went through these early years of developing madness, attempting, unsuccessfully, to mature and to find work. He became progressively more remote and dejected, he took menial jobs which he could not hold on to. Unrecognised and untreated symptoms were distressing and probably damaging to him and for the family. An individual with early schizophrenia is very frightened, has moments of real terror and outbursts of anger. We trailed around surgeries looking for help, accepting such statements as, 'he will grow out of it', and, 'it is just a difficult adolescence', because we wanted it to be so, while deep down knowing that something was very wrong. Carers feel impotent, powerless and desperate. It is a very difficult time for all because they do not know what questions to ask.

For our son, I see these early years as wasted. They might have made a difference to the outcome of the illness. The fear professionals have of labelling a young person with such a dreadful diagnosis as schizophrenia is understandable, but their reluctance also reinforces the myths which surround the illness. It is not uncommon for the term psychosis to be used instead of schizophrenia. Whatever the term, earlier intervention is vital particularly for the first episode, and any subsequent relapses: the professionals must listen and hear what the carers and users are saying. I believe that individuals have a right to know what is wrong with them, the treatment and how it works, and that to prevaricate is to patronise and disempower the individual.

The advent of chlorpromazine was a very great step forward, liberating many people who were previously condemned to live with their voices and fear, but it did not work for everybody and for many, it produced frightening side-effects or no benefit at all. The newer, more specific neuroleptics must be the first-line choice and, if prescribed, could be another great step forward. Their better profile may prevent patients stopping their medication and so reduce the deteriorating effects of relapse, improving the image of schizophrenia for the next generation. This would certainly be empowering. It is only recently that talking therapies like cognitive behavioural therapy and the positive idea of partnership between the patient, carers and professionals have been recognised as possible. The Mental Health Foundation paper, *Pull Yourself Together* (2000), found that acceptance and involvement by professionals was felt by users to be the most empowering aspect of care and treatment, while medication, though important, was rated second overall.

Our son often said that he used me as a sounding board.

However, I also know that he thought at times that I was poisoning him. Empowerment is about supporting people by keeping respect for their dignity and by staying honest and representing the real world, while recognising and acknowledging the individual's own distorted view.

Remember, it is the illness which you see, not the individual. It is important always to keep your patient informed about what you are doing, and why. Do not assume that he or she will not understand, or does not need to.

Both users and carers need courage and determination in order to achieve the best possible deal. I have been in contact with hundreds of families over the years and the majority I have found tend to be normal ordinary people whose lives have been turned upside down by the illness. What I can assure you, is that the appearance of schizophrenia may well create a dysfunctional family. I am still in contact with a few families with carers in their eighties, who years ago, were told that they caused their child's illness and who still feel that label.

I was once told that it would be important for me to stay well and to gauge the contact I had with my son. Achieving balance is very individual. Many carers do break down or move away because they cannot cope. It must be a part of the work of the care teams to assess the carer's needs and provide for them. All efforts which may lead to self-empowerment for users and carers need to be encouraged and supported, provided the individual is not set up to fail.

Historical developments

Society today is about individuals. Psychiatry has come a long way from when people were incarcerated in the old mental hospitals with their mixed populations of people diagnosed as having a mental illness or learning disability, or considered to be socially inadequate. Patients had little identity outside these hospitals and were largely forgotten by society. I see the emptying of the mental hospitals as the first step towards the recovery of identity for these people, but the Utopian idea that, given normal surroundings all would recover, was very misconceived. The result was that thousands disappeared into the community without trace, families concealed their relatives from the public because of the stigma. Schizophrenia was a 'skeleton in the cupboard illness', and it still is today in some sections of our community.

The old 'bins' and their outdated treatment and image have been slow to pass. Hospital staff had to be re-trained and a less custodial flavour cultivated. Many of these patients living in the community were still easily recognised by their ill-fitting clothes, restless movements and shakes produced by their medication, confirming for the public the image of mental patients being a danger. It is not possible to be a part of a community if you cannot afford a pint in a pub. Appearance and financial constraints inhibited rehabilitation and disempower service users. The mentally ill have been moved around to meet the needs of society and this has been concealed under the umbrella of 'normalisation'. The real problem has been the optimism with which the move has been done. Academics debated the social and biological theories of mental illness, while the patients sat in poverty. 'Health' saw its role as diagnosing and stabilising individuals on medication and discharging them to 'the community' where 'social care' expected them to lead normal lives. Today, health and social care bodies have a duty to work together and have recognised the benefits of this. Hopefully, this will bring forward a culture which is about involvement, sharing, supporting; in short, empowering.

So what is needed for empowerment?

Users and carers ask for information, information enlightens and empowers: without it we are all plunged into superstition and fear. They need information about the condition, its treatments, side-effects and likely outcomes, shared on a need to know basis and to be put in touch with local voluntary agencies providing appropriate information and support and contact with others in the same position. Users must be seen as people with individual needs and their care must be planned holistically, with the involvement and agreement of all those contributing, including the user and carer. The benefits of teamwork lie in the diversity of ideas and the safety of shared knowledge and involvement. Carers must be trained to care appropriately and be supported to do so.

Sharing coping strategies and alternative ways of dealing with difficult situations are vital. Carers may give up if unsupported. The burden is heavy and for their life time. Many carers talk about a bereavement from which they cannot move on.

Professionals need to guard against loss of family support to the users. Severe mental illness is too serious an illness to be helped by the merely sympathetic approach. People effected need to get to grips with it as soon as possible. It is still the case that 50% of individuals with a severe mental illness are discharged to the family home, and the bulk of individual care is provided by family carers. Secrecy must no longer be justified on the false premise of confidentiality. The professionals who gain the confidence of the individual empower him/her through inclusion in all aspects of the care partnership and its planning.

Rationing of care is unacceptable, and the best treatments must be made available. I believe that we all have a duty to the future generations of people who will develop a severe mental illness, to do things better.

Key points

✺ Individuals with mental illness lose rights when they are compulsorily admitted. Although this is disempowering, carers may welcome the opportunity for rest and the start of treatment. Rehabilitation and renewed independence are important aspects of empowerment following detention. Some people have been left, untreated, to deteriorate at home.

✺ A diagnosis of schizophrenia results in various forms of social exclusion, but may enable the individual and his/her carers to obtain information, explanations and support.

✺ Both service users and carers are stigmatised by wider society. Following the closure of large institutions, problems for people with schizophrenia have continued, with isolation in the community and limited finances. In addition, research has found that some service users are 'discriminated against by their families'.

✺ There are many issues of control in relation to people with schizophrenia, with opposing views, particularly related to interventions without individuals' consent. Some control measures are excessive. It is disempowering for service users to be labelled 'aggressive', and feel they can never lose their temper. If control is seen as appropriate, it must always respect the individual, and be based on training and skilled interventions.

⌘ Factors of crucial importance include early interventions for individuals with schizophrenia, the professional-client relationship and the use of the newer psychoactive drugs.

⌘ One study found that professionals' acceptance and facilitation of client participation was considered by service users to be 'the most empowering aspect of care and treatment'. Factors necessary for empowerment include partnership approaches, adequate information for both service users and carers, and involving them in the planning of care.

⌘ An individual's schizophrenia may cause considerable problems, including threatening behaviour, resulting in carers' disempowerment. Professionals need to listen to, assess and meet the needs of relatives, who provide most of the care, and who can feel 'impotent, powerless and desperate' casualties among us, to further our understanding of whatever condition besets us — freely, with dignity, and without shame.

Reference

Mental Health Foundation (2000) *Pull Yourself Together.* Mental Health Foundation, London

13

Making empowerment a reality: a personal account

Caroline Byrt, Marian Weeks, Richard Byrt

This account is in memory of our father, Mr WH Byrt. It outlines ways in which staff on Abergavenny ward, Nevill Hall Hospital, empowered both Dad and ourselves, as his closest relatives, during the last seven weeks of his life. We feel that, in view of his concern for other people, our father would be happy for our account to appear in this book.

Throughout his ninety-one years, our father showed incredible courage and determination. Despite many difficulties and hardships, he always retained his highly original sense of humour. A loving husband and father, he always worked incredibly hard and had a variety of interesting jobs as a gardener, as well as work in a mental health hospital and with homeless people. Dad held very radical ideas for the time in relation to people living with mental health problems or homelessness. In World War II, he served in the Royal Engineers and later, in particular, in the Royal Army Medical Corps. He was a prisoner of war for over three years in Germany and Eastern Europe.

In his eighties, our father faced two further difficulties with his customary courage: the death of his wife (our mother) and the onset of multi-infarct dementia. In addition, the deafness which he had experienced since early adulthood, became progressively worse. In July, 2000, Dad sustained a fractured neck and upper shaft of femur following a fall, and was admitted to Nevill Hall Hospital.

Initial impressions

The initial impressions which a client/patient or visitor receives from any health service can be either empowering or disempowering:

> *When a patient enters... a health facility, communication begins long before he meet a member of staff. Everything speaks — the location, the buildings, the gardens, the colour of the walls, the furniture and the faces of the*

*people he passes. The messages he receives may be: 'This
is a hospital, go away unless you are sick...' or it may be
'this is a friendly place...'.*

(Jones, 1988, p. 158)

On admission to the accident and emergency department, and later to
Abergavenny ward, attempts were made to make our father and the
relative accompanying him feel welcome. This was despite the fact
that both the department and the ward were busy. From the time of
his admission, staff endeavoured to work in partnership with Dad
and his relatives. The importance of such partnership has been
emphasised in recent Department of Health policies (DoH, 1999;
2000). An important component of partnership is clear communication
from professionals, including the willingness to listen to clients/
patients and their informal carers and to consider their perspectives.
Staff in both Accident and Emergency and Abergavenny ward took
careful note of our account of our father's communication difficulties
related to his lack of hearing and multi-infarct dementia. Staff
continued our usual methods of communication with Dad through
touch, gestures and the use of written communications.

Lack of information has been found to be a major source of
dissatisfaction and complaint in both accident and emergency
departments (Audit Commission, 1996; Lau, 2000) and acute services
(Health Service Ombudsman for England, 2000; Rogers *et al*, 2000).
In relation to our father, reasons for delay were explained. In addition,
without being asked, a staff nurse provided the accompanying relative
with details of guest houses so that he could stay locally overnight.

Dad's nursing and medical care continued, without delays, on
his transfer to Abergavenny ward. A staff nurse undertook a detailed
assessment and explained, as necessary, the reasons for the various
questions which she asked.

Our father's physical environment and care

The importance of the physical environment in patient/client care is
increasingly recognised (Bechtel, 1997; Lawson and Phiri, 2000).
Dad was admitted to a light, well-decorated side room with a very
pleasant view of trees and flowers. He was able to remain in this
room throughout his stay on the ward. Nevill Hall Hospital is set in
outstandingly beautiful grounds in what was once a country estate of

The Marquis of Abergavenny. Abergavenny ward itself has a small garden with seats for the use of both patients and their visitors. In addition, the 'Branching Out Appeal' has initiated horticultural projects for the benefit of patients. Work includes the development of the grounds, incorporating an orchard, an area of woodland and a sensory garden with access for people using wheelchairs (Branching Out Appeal, undated).

> To treat the patient, relative or significant other as one would want to be treated, or how one would want our nearest and dearest to be treated and cared for while in hospital.
>
> Our philosophy is that patients or relatives should be empowered to make informed choices about their care and treatment while in hospital. For empowerment to occur, staff need to be educated and use evidence-based research practice, in order to enhance competency and efficiency while maintaining the focus on the patient's needs.
>
> There must be an open and honest relationship between the patient, their family and professionals to engender feelings of security in the practice of care and the system of its delivery.
>
> Empowerment is a means of supporting both patients and relatives who are given 'permission' to ask questions, question decisions and participate in their care. Staff efforts to inform and enable the patient and relative will help them to feel a sense of control in an unfamiliar situation.
>
> Security and a sense of control will help make empowerment a reality, not just a concept.

Box 13.1: Philosophy of Abergavenny ward, Marian Weeks, ward sister

Efficient, competent and sensitive nursing care can contribute to the satisfaction and empowerment of patients/clients and their visitors (Martin, 1998; Rogers *et al*, 2000). Indeed, without such care, it is questionable whether such empowerment is possible. Unsatisfactory care, and in some cases, considerable neglect of terminally ill patients' basic needs, have been reported (Rogers *et al*, 2000). In contrast, efforts were made to ensure the meeting of our father's physical needs and comfort. While there were effective interventions from nursing, medical and physiotherapy staff, in general, there were also attempts to ensure unnecessary disturbance and discomfort from procedures. There was attention to details which were important to Dad and to ourselves. These included his room being kept spotlessly clean, fresh attractive bed linen and a well-designed, easily adjustable bed. As our father's physical health worsened, his pyjamas were replaced with reasonably attractive gowns which were easy to remove, with the minimum of disturbance. The knowledge that our father received a high standard of nursing care and was clean and comfortable was of great importance to us, and is reflected in research on informal carers' views (Royal College of Physicians and College of Health, 1998).

Communication

During his stay on Abergavenny ward, our father found it increasingly hard to communicate, especially verbally. Difficulty in communication can be a source of considerable isolation, frustration and feelings of disempowerment to patients (Barnes and Ward, 2000; Royal College of Physicians and College of Health, 1998). Staff made efforts to understand Dad's communication problems and the consequences for him. Both family and staff continued to communicate through touch, gestures and writing clearly on his whiteboard. The hospital chaplain visited whenever necessary and provided additional support.

Rogers *et al* (2000) report from their study of relatives of people with terminal illnesses:

> *Much of the dissatisfaction with hospital-based care... related to the way hospital staff communicated with patients... seventeen respondents reported difficulties in getting information concerning the patient's condition and likely prognosis from hospital staff.*

> (Rogers *et al*, 2000, p. 770)

In contrast, despite our father's considerable communication difficulties, staff endeavoured to give him information about his fracture and his nursing care and treatment.

Teasdale (1998) refers to the importance of nurses enabling advocacy by both patients/clients and their informal carers. We were not 'easy' relatives in our attempts to advocate for Dad and our many questions. However, staff listened to our views, involved us in decision making and invited us to a ward round concerned with our father's care and treatment. Our own views were carefully considered and taken into account. Many relatives of patients in hospital have described lack of adequate information (Health Service Ombudsman, 2000; Royal College of Physicians and College of Health, 1998). On Abergavenny ward, we were given information clearly, honestly and sensitively. On one occasion when this was not possible, an apology and explanation was given. Decisions about whether or not to resuscitate, and Dad's likely wishes, were carefully discussed with us, as were plans for his future care and treatment. This included surgeons' information and explanations about decisions not to carry out orthopaedic surgery.

Nursing staff enabled us to communicate with our father through the things which he had always liked or enjoyed. We were grateful that there were no restrictions on items which we could bring into his room, and it was possible to give this a homely touch. We looked with Dad at his photograph albums, which included his most treasured snaps and a record of his past and his achievements. Some studies have found that sadly, the present and past identities of older people are not always appreciated or recognised in health services (Downs, 2000; Small *et al*, 1998).

Our father was always a very keen and highly skilled gardener throughout his life. This was reflected in the many pot plants and cut flowers in his room, including ones which he could smell, as well as see. Among these was an orchid: one of his favourite plants. The room also included a variety or objects d'art, of meaning to Dad, and a colourful mobile.

As our father became progressively more ill, verbal communication, using the whiteboard, became increasingly difficult. It was possible to communicate through touch. Dad often squeezed our hands, and was able to do so until his level of consciousness decreased a few hours before he died.

The staff empowered us to participate in our father's care whenever we wished. In particular, they enabled us to play a pro-active role in contributing to his comfort in the last days and hours of his life. Dad particularly appeared to enjoy his mouth care, and it was important for us to share this activity with him. At times, he also appeared to enjoy the smell of citrus pot pourri.

Staff's awareness of our needs

Staff were very aware of our own needs. The domestic staff frequently gave us cups of coffee and we were offered food at times when it was difficult for us to get to the hospital restaurant. It was made clear that we could visit at any time, and that we could stay on the ward at night whenever we wished. Nursing staff went out of their way to enable us to do this. When our father was particularly ill, they provided chairs, pillows and blankets so that we could stay with him overnight.

On one occasion, when one of us was particularly tired and distressed, a senior staff nurse suggested taking a break in the hospital grounds. Quiet reflection by the lily pond, under the shadow of the nearby Sugar Loaf Mountain, was of great benefit at this time!

The approachability of all staff was empowering, both to our father and ourselves. We had the impression of a team of professionals who got on well with each other and with patients and their visitors. At the same time, it was very clear who was in charge of the ward. The ward sister was highly visible and made herself available to both Dad and ourselves. By his bed, was a brief note of welcome to the ward, with the name of the ward sister and primary nurse and an explanation that they could be contacted with particular queries.

'Dying in the best possible way'

> *Dying and death are a natural part of human life. By an appropriate death is meant the death an individual would choose if it was possible to choose: 'dying in the best possible way.'*
>
> (Sahlberg-Blom *et al*, 2000, p. 296, quoting Weisman, 1988)

Abergavenny ward staff enabled our father to die 'in the best possible way': peacefully and with dignity. They made it easy for us to be with Dad at this time. As usual, they ensured that his needs for comfort were met, with as little disturbance as possible. They also ensured the meeting of our own needs during our father's last hours and immediately after he died. When this occurred, nursing staff made themselves available and brought us tea and biscuits, but were also sensitive to our needs for space and to be on our own. The following day, sister spent time with us in her office and enabled us to collect and donate items of our father's property, as he would have wished.

'Patient and carer empowerment' can be a cliché. On Abergavenny ward it was a reality.

Key points

⌘ Two of the authors outline aspects of their father's life, achievements, and the care he received in the last weeks of his life.

⌘ The initial welcome, other first impressions of the health service, and the opportunity to work in partnership with professionals were important in the experience described.

⌘ The individual and his relatives were empowered through the maintenance of high standards of care, attention to the physical environment, including cleanliness, the giving of information and other aspects of communication.

⌘ The ward philosophy, in relation to empowerment, is outlined. The ward sister was highly visible and available to patients and relatives. A welcoming message gave clear information about the name of the ward sister and primary nurse.

⌘ The need for imaginative communication with service users who are seriously ill, using a variety of methods, and involving all five senses, is illustrated.

⌘ The authors' positive experiences are contrasted with research findings of poor care and communication experienced by many service users and their carers.

⌘ Staff enabled the relatives to advocate for their father, visit at any time, and be involved in his care. They also ensured that relatives' needs for rest and refreshment were met. Considerable flexibility was allowed in enabling their father to keep plants and other items, of value to him, in his room on the ward.

⌘ Staff enabled him to die peacefully and with dignity, and also met the needs of the relatives at this time.

References

Audit Commission (1996) *By Accident or Design. Improving Accident and Emergency Services in England and Wales*. HMSO, London

Barnes MP, Ward AB (2000) *Textbook of Rehabilitation Medicine*. Oxford University Press, Oxford

Bechtel RB (1997) *Environment and Behaviour. An Introduction*. Sage Publications,Thousand Oaks, California

Branching Out Appeal (Undated) Nevill Hall Millennium Garden Project. Leaflet

Department of Health (1999) *Patient and Public Involvement in the New NHS*. DoH, London: September

Department of Health (2000) *The NHS Plan. A Plan for Investment. A Plan for Reform*. DoH, London

Downs M (2000) Dementia in a socio-cultural context: an idea whose time has come. *Ageing and Society* **20**(3): 369–75

Health Service Ombudsman For England (2000) *Second Report for Session 1999–2000. Part 1. Summaries of Investigations Completed, October, 1999–March, 2000*. HMSO, London

Jones K (1988) *Experience in Mental Health. Community Care and Social Policy*. Sage Publications, London

Lau K (2000) Can communication skills workshops for emergency department doctors improve patient satisfaction? *J Accid Emerg Med* **17**(4): 251–3

Lawson B, Phiri M (2000) Room for improvement. *Health Service J*, 20 January: 24–7

Martin GW (1998) Empowerment of dying patients: the strategies and barriers to patient autonomy. *J Adv Nurs* **28**(4): 737–44

Rogers A, Karlsen S, Addington-Hall J (2000) All the services were excellent. It is when the human element comes in that things go wrong: dissatisfaction with hospital care in the last year of life. *J Adv Nurs* **31**(4): 768–74

Royal College of Physicians and College of Health (1998) *Stroke Rehabilitation, Patient and Carer Views. A Report From the Intercollegiate Working Party for Stroke*. Royal College of Physicians of London, London: November

Sahlberg-Blom E, Ternestedt B-M, Johansson J-E (2000) Patient participation in decision making at the end of life as seen by a close relative. *Nurs Ethics* **7**(4): 296–311

Small JA, Geldart K, Gutman, G, Clarke Scott MA (1998) The discourse of self in dementia. *Ageing and Society* **18**: 291–316.

Teasdale K (1998) *Advocacy in Health Care*. Blackwell Science, Oxford

14

The effects of being turned into a clown for the amusement of 'professionals'

'Sue'

My first fifteen years of 'psychiatric' life was spent on the same acute ward. I was a regular' customer' and spent long periods of time there. Indeed, I got quite attached to the place. Staff came and went until I had been there longer than most of the staff. The other patients were mostly short stay so I would make friends, and then they would be discharged. After a while some of the discharges would be re-admitted. During my time in this acute ward there seemed to be a group of four patients who were the 'regulars'. Each of us had strong reputations on the unit. We were 'in charge', we controlled the 'smoke room'. If another patient picked an argument with one of us then they may as well give up smoking because we made life extremely unpleasant for them.

The four of us had our own specific traits to our illnesses, which must have made it hard for everybody else when we were in together, which was quite often. As I look back, it was our way of coping with an unfair and uncaring system.

I had been shaped into a two-sided personality. My high side made me the joker, with a very exaggerated sense of humour. I did everything to exaggerate my feelings like wearing bright shirts, which I would change several times a day. Staff encouraged me to do this.

Over the years my illness changed, the peaks lessened but no one, including me, seemed to notice. I had built up a reputation for myself that the staff, the doctors and whole unit expected. I knew no different, and I honestly believed that I was that reputation. I was encouraged to be that reputation. I used to walk around the unit and everybody knew me. From cleaners to office staff, and they all saw me in one light. My consultant actively encouraged me to behave in a high manner, and I used to shout nicknames I had given him down the corridors and he seemed to enjoy it. In this way he used to encourage me. I used to draw in the dust on his car but instead of getting annoyed he would put it down to a symptom of my highness. My Grandma said, 'They're turning "Sue" into a clown!' and it seemed they were doing this for their own amusement. I had no control and developed my behaviours to please the staff's expectations of me.

When I became low I would shrivel up into my bedroom away from the public eye. This over-familiar relationship I had developed with the consultant worked against me, and he did not take my mental health seriously. Over the years I had told staff about thoughts being put into my head but because of this relationship, I did not want him to think I'd gone 'loopy'. When these thoughts changed from thoughts to voices, I could not seem to explain and never told him. I struggled on alone and I think that even if I had told him he would have given me so little time that I would not have been able to express myself properly.

Most of the time the only chance you got to see your consultant was in a two-minute slot at ward round. In ward round there were usually three to four nurses from the ward, two student doctors or nurses, a social worker, registrar, any other professionals and the consultant himself. If I was 'high' it was great, almost a ready made stage to perform on. Staff preferred me in a high mood and actively egged me on, by saying things like, 'that's a happy shirt today', or, 'tell us that joke you said earlier'.

When low, ward rounds were intimidating and frightening, too much to bear. I felt that I could not speak my feelings in front of all those people.

I feel that when my illness was at its most severe, acute care was the only option offered to me. Although not ideal, it served its purpose, but, as I became more settled, acute 'care' did me untold damage.

Moving to rehabilitation has really helped. At last I can see the person that I really am. The staff treat me in a more realistic way and I have no image to keep up! Instead, they are trying to find ways for me to live with my illness. There are a lot of positive things to do to regain my confidence and true standing in the outside world. I have joined a group called Remit, which is a college for people who have had mental health problems. I do computers and creative writing classes. I enjoy both so much that I have bought a computer and also write at home as a hobby.

I have also started doing voluntary work in a charity shop. I enjoy it very much as it is nice to have something in my life that is completely away from my mental health reputation

Since I have been in this rehabilitation service I can at last see the possibility of leading a 'normal life' again.

Key points

⌘ The 'psychiatric career' of clients is often longer than the professionals who are caring for them, and their experience of the inpatient environment spans the twenty-four-hour period throughout an inpatient stay. The author was admitted to the same acute ward over fifteen years. During this time, she became well known in the mental health unit. She acquired a reputation for being 'high', which was actively encouraged by staff.

⌘ 'Sue' was able to develop a complete 24/7 picture of the service being provided, which enabled her to assess and compare the quality of individual staff interventions.

⌘ 'Sue' is a survivor of the system but her survival has little to do with the first fifteen years spent in an acute ward. A move to rehabilitation services has been helpful. Staff do not expect the author to conform to a particular image, but attempt to find ways to enable her to live with her illness. Further education and voluntary work are very enjoyable, and the author can 'see the possibility of leading a normal life again'.

15

Involving users in clinical governance: the Somerset experience

Nicky Pearson and Martin Carter

Whose service is it anyway?

The National Health Service has entered a new millennium and its second half century. Those working in it and using it in 1948 would scarcely recognise the NHS of today. Thankfully, much has changed for the better. The range and quality of care available now would seem little short of miraculous to its early pioneers. It is not just medical, pharmaceutical and surgical interventions which have taken quantum leaps forward. The way that we now plan and configure services, work with partner agencies, and see the role of the NHS, have also changed beyond recognition. For the first time in its history, the NHS is finally in the forefront of health improvement — becoming, at last, a genuine national health service rather than merely a sickness or remedial one.

But, some vital things have not changed, none more important than the principles upon which the NHS was conceived and founded. Public funding and ownership of the NHS remains its most important and defining characteristic. In particular, what is changing rapidly (particularly over the past decade), and for the better, is the dynamic of the relationship between patients and the practitioner. Patients can now expect to be far more involved in all aspects of the service rather than being the passive recipients of its care and treatment. Professionals are beginning to accept that they have a central role in helping patients — who have been somewhat disenfranchised, even patronised, until now — in understanding and making the most of their active role as partners in their health care. Most patients are well aware that they have rights within the health system. More emphasis now has to be placed on their responsibilities. In the same way that clinicians cannot, and should not, be expected to take full responsibility for the totality of their patients' welfare, so patients have to accept that to be influential in that relationship, they have a responsibility to be active partners. All patients (and professionals) are individuals, and, therefore, different. This means that there is a spectrum of relationships or partnerships that will exist, determined by how informed and assertive patients are, and the degree of readiness that the clinicians exhibit in embracing this new dynamic (Hogg, 1999).

Citizens have every right not just to see for themselves how well the NHS is discharging its publicly funded duties, but also to have an influential role in the way it goes about its work. If clinical governance is about ensuring that the best possible care is provided, in the best and most appropriate and timely way for each individual, then service users, and potential or future service users, have every right to expect meaningful involvement in the way that the NHS operates now and in the future.

The NHS has been pursuing the holy grail of excellence for all four decades. Relatively recently, we have had medical audit, clinical audit, clinical effectiveness initiatives, total quality management and quality assurance. All of these have been worthy and, to greater or lesser degrees, successful. Clinical governance — and its place within overall controls assurance frameworks — has made these aspirations much more real, meaningful and potentially powerful.

One of the key things which distinguishes clinical governance from its precursors is the active and visible involvement of patients and the public in the core business of the NHS — delivering the best possible health care for the UK within the constraints of what the public is prepared collectively to pay for the Department of Health (1998). A useful working definition of clinical governance is 'putting patients at the very centre of their care'.

Clearly, high profile failures and controversies such as those surrounding the Bristol Royal Infirmary inquiry and the Harold Shipman case have propelled this issue into the limelight and into the public consciousness.

There is a danger — real or perceived — that the new emphasis on clinical governance could act as a barrier to innovation within the NHS. Health professionals are somewhat divided in their perceptions of clinical governance. Many do see it simply as a policing or regulatory function, but as a genuine drive towards excellence, the sharing of good practice and a real support mechanism to deliver care of the highest quality. Others are less convinced and believe that the high priority of Government ministers and the NHS to establish clinical governance is a knee-jerk reaction to some high profile failures. This suspicion, even mistrust, of the motivation for clinical governance, could hold back progress or reduce the pace of change and innovation. Professionals are less likely to take risks or become involved in research if there is a danger of controversy or sanction.

Involving service users and the public in clinical governance should have a positive influence in this respect. The drive for effective clinical governance does, in large measure, reflect public opinion and concern about standards of care, treatment and safety. By and large, people are perfectly capable of making their own decisions about the levels of risk or discomfort that they are prepared to accept in health care, as they do in other areas of life, and which they think should be acceptable to most people. What matters of course, is that they are able to participate in the right way. Bringing patients, the public and professionals closer together through clinical governance arrangements should serve to make the partnership between these various parties more equal and meaningful.

Making clinical governance work for patients

What does clinical governance mean to people? To the average person on the street (if such a person actually exists) the concept is probably quite simplistic and straightforward, getting it right first time, every time, with no mistakes — achieving the outcome that is most important to the patient. To health professionals the concept is more complex and is as much to do with health systems and the environment of care as the delivery of health services.

If clinical governance is to work for patients, they must function as partners (albeit, not always equal ones) with those responsible for their care and treatment and understand their role in that relationship. By definition, partnerships cannot be imposed; they have to be built, forged and sustained.

The NHS is already putting the infrastructure in place to support this concept. Clinical governance is now recognised as an essential component part of the care process, rather than a luxury or optional extra (DoH, 1998; DoH, 1999; DoH, 2001). Health authorities and NHS trusts have appointed senior people to take responsibility for this area of work. Primary care trusts (PCTs) are addressing the clinical governance agenda with vigour, as are the majority of health professionals. The Government has augmented this increased emphasis on clinical governance through the establishment of the Commission for Health Improvement and the National Institute for Clinical Effectiveness (NICE).

Inevitably, the depth and quality of user and public participation efforts around the country is extremely variable — perhaps mirroring the unacceptable variations in access and quality of care, which have created the necessity for this development.

There are few, if any, ready-made tool kits or made-to-measure solutions for how to involve successfully patients and local people in planning and delivering NHS services. There are many right ways to do this, just as there are many wrong ways.

This chapter contains two real life examples of an approach that has worked for us in Somerset and which could be remodelled or adapted for use elsewhere. We do not profess these examples to be perfect or right for everyone. They do, we hope, provide useful food for thought and pointers to the potential benefits and pitfalls that come from constructive engagement with patients and the public.

Involving users in service planning

Firstly, what do we mean by 'planning?'. The dictionary defines planning as a method or procedure for doing something; to arrange beforehand, or to produce a scheme or design (Davidson *et al*, 1989). Ideally, plans begin with two popular clichés: the blank sheet of paper and the open mind. In reality, we plan within constraints and predeterminations. We cannot, for example, plan a health system which would cost double the entire gross national product, even though it would be quite possible to do so.

An important early step in the process of participation is to ensure that our partners (in this case patients and local populations) are aware of the parameters within which we have to plan, and the constraints upon what we can actually plan for. In this way, we prepare the ground for progressing from participation to empowerment. Empowerment is a slightly contentious issue and beyond what we wish to address here, although high quality involvement processes most certainly have a significant role to play in any project with the longer-term aim of empowerment.

Involving the community in all aspects of care delivery: the Somerset health panels

This case study describes a system pioneered and developed in Somerset in 1993 and conducted regularly ever since for consulting with, and involving, the wider local population in decisions about the health care.

The panels take the form of focus groups and have, as of Autumn 2000, been run eighteen times.

In Somerset, giving maximum voice and influence to patients and local people, with regard to their own care and decisions about the configuration and delivery of NHS services, is embodied in an overall strategy for user and public participation in the NHS. It has been a high priority for Somerset Health Authority for several years and has been one of the top five objectives within our corporate contracts/performance agreements with the NHS executive for at least five years.

Just as the NHS has been changing and evolving, so has our approach to the health panels and the way that they have been run and used.

Originally, the panels were staged in eight locations throughout Somerset, three times a year. They were later reconfigured to be run twice a year in ten locations. In early 2000, it was agreed to reconfigure the panels again so that they are now held in twelve locations, twice each year. This ensures that three panels in each round are held within each of Somerset's four primary care trust (PCT) areas. This allows PCT comparative analysis to be undertaken and the report is now written in a way that reflects this. These changes have allowed more thoroughness and influence to be incorporated into the process, and ensure that the panels are held at the optimum time within our business planning cycle.

The mechanics of running the panels are as follows:

Stage 1 — what do we want to know?

Around two to three months before each round of panel meetings, a range of interested parties are invited to submit proposals for panel discussions. These partners include senior health authority staff and non-executives, the community health council (CHC), colleagues from Somerset social services, the county's four primary care groups, local NHS trusts and the local medical committee (LMC).

Proposals are debated with a final decision as to which topics should be discussed being taken by either the health authority's policy and performance board — a high level health authority/PCG/NHS Trust body — or the health authority board itself.

Stage 2 — developing the topic guide

A facilitator is appointed for the health panels, and information about the topics to be discussed is gathered before meetings take place. A topic guide is produced by all those with a stake in the issues under discussion. This usually comprises the health authority, CHC, LMC, PCGs and original proposers of topics. The facilitator, is also heavily involved, and care is taken to ensure that the topic guide is as balanced as possible, setting out clearly the agenda, and terms of reference. Panel members are encouraged to discuss the topics for consideration with families and friends.

Stage 3 — recruitment and organisation

Panel members are recruited by independent recruiters according to a sample based on a quota, derived mainly from census data with the aim of finding a representative cross section of local communities. The quota is based upon age, sex, educational level and number of dependent children under the age of fifteen. Up to twelve panel members attend each discussion and serve for three rounds of panels. At any given panel meeting, there will be one-third of panellists attending for their first time, one-third for their second time and a third for their third and final time. Recruiters provide information to potential panel members to ensure that they understand what they are being invited to take part in, and why. Recruitment is done door-to-door, rather than by post or over the telephone, which could introduce bias into the system.

Suitable venues in each location are identified, visited if necessary, and booked by a senior member of the health authority's staff. Meetings are held in the early evening and every effort is made to ensure that disabled access is available, together with tape-loop systems and any other facilities if needed. Panel members are paid £10.00 for attending and are also reimbursed travel costs if necessary.

Stage 4 — holding the meetings

Panel meetings are always run by an experienced independent facilitator and can be observed by up to two interested parties, who are instructed not to make comments or become involved in discussions. Usually, two or three topics are discussed and panels can be asked to make shadow decisions on issues being debated within the local health community, or list priorities in order of preference. The meetings are tape recorded and transcribed so that a summative analysis can be carried out and a report prepared. Original tapes and transcripts are kept but are not shared outside the health authority, to maintain confidentiality and guarantee anonymity to panel members. The report is then presented to a meeting of the health authority board in public session and debated.

Stage 5 — feedback and publicity

The report is shared with relevant partners and sent to all participants before being discussed by the health authority. News releases and other publicity materials are produced, which are also shared. The panels have been subject to considerable amounts of local and national publicity, including features and documentaries on national television and radio. Each round of panel meetings leads to considerable amounts of local newspaper and radio coverage, although the media are not permitted to attend the panel meetings themselves.

Since 1993, the panels have discussed a wide range of issues, including:

- the targeting of resources (eg. health visitors) at areas of highest need
- timing of the opening of satellite renal dialysis units
- the adoption of a scoring system to prioritise patients on waiting lists
- whether access to the voluntary ambulance car service should be reduced
- availability of incontinence pads on the NHS
- how the public can best influence PCGs
- the most appropriate setting for follow-up routine cancer care
- the availability of Viagra on the NHS
- the use of alternative therapies
- confidential drug services for under-sixteens

- using NHS Direct as the sole gateway to NHS services.

The panels project is also being assessed by an independent researcher as part of an academic study. Part of that study included an analysis of whether or not panels' views had influenced health authority decision making or actions. This analysis shows that in more than 70% of cases, the views expressed by the panels had had a direct impact on service planning and/or delivery. For example, panels recommended that the health authority should provide a greater number of antenatal visits for new mothers than were recommended nationally and that had been provided locally, up to that point. Those views were listened to and acted upon.

The study was not, however, entirely positive or complementary and highlighted areas where improvements could be made. In particular, more than 60% of the county's GPs were, at that time, either unaware of the health panels or did not consider them to be worthwhile.

Over the past couple of years, attempts have been made to address this. These efforts are ongoing and should be strengthened further by the greater involvement of Somerset's PCTs in the panel's process. PCTs have been extremely supportive. They see the panels as an excellent way of accessing local opinion and involving the wider community in healthcare planning and decision-making. They have made particular use of panels in determining their own input to the county's health improvement programme and primary care investment plans. The PCTs have embraced the panel's model to the extent that they are now making a financial contribution to the cost of running them.

In a recent round of panel meetings, the format of the panel discussions was changed. Rather than asking panels to reach decisions on specific issues, they were engaged in a more open discussion on areas of inequality in health, with particular focus on heart disease, teenage conception and childhood accidents. This was done to inform the latest version of the county's health improvement plan, and has had a considerable impact on plans for future action and, consequently, investment.

In this way, considerably more emphasis was given to the qualitative data gathered from the panels. In the past, the results have been a mixture of quantitative and qualitative research data. In addition, a specialist health and healthcare evaluation manager from within the health authority has been conducting the detailed analysis of the panel discussions.

Use of the panels is now being extended further to partner agencies, such as PCTs, social services staff and NHS trusts. Topics of specific relevance to one or more of the county's PCTs have already been included in recent rounds of panel discussions.The panels are seen as being particularly useful to health service planners and their partners on two broad fronts:

❖ Identifying and scoping issues of particular importance or relevance to specific geographical communities within Somerset.

❖ Influencing county-wide issues, such as prescribing and development of health improvement programmes (incorporating the county's community care plan).

The following quotations are from former health panel members responding to questions from an independent source, a BBC television interviewer:

> *They should take notice of us — we pay, we make our contribution towards it and we are the shareholders of the National Health Service and they should take notice of us.*

> *These (the panels) are marvellous. We get a chance to hear other people's views. You realise that young people have got completely different ideas to older ones. As you get older you get more mature, perhaps more vehement. It's a great idea — really good.*

> *I think they are excellent. I mean, we have seen some of the feedback, we have seen some of the results of some of the previous panels. I think it's a good idea for the public to be able to give their point of view, rather than someone high up who doesn't know what the general public feels, and this a cross section — all age groups and all sorts of types of people and what have you, it's not just one type of person giving their opinion.*

Involving users — lessons for practice

There are already many volumes written on this subject — many considerably better researched and informed than it is possible for us to be at this stage. However, the processes undertaken, as outlined above and within this book as a whole, have provided a number of lessons for us at local level, which we are happy to share.

Decide why you want user participation before embarking upon it

There is little point devoting time, energy and resources unless you are clear what influence you are prepared to allow users and the public to have. If a decision has already been made, or there is no intention to undertake participation in a meaningful way, do not raise false expectations through participation exercises. It needs to be clear from the outset, what level of engagement you are seeking and why. Sometimes involvement of users is an information-giving process, sometimes a listening exercise and occasionally, genuinely empowering, with users having a direct impact on service planning and delivery. Once it is clear what level of engagement is desired, it becomes much easier to select the right method(s) and to evaluate the outcome.

Involve users and the public in planning the participation process itself

This is not always possible, but has significant benefits in terms of increased credibility if it can be achieved. It can be surprising how innovative people can be and how much service planners take for granted! This is also helpful in overcoming understandable but sometimes embarrassing, or even damaging, *faux pas*, such as inviting people with mobility problems to a meeting at a venue with no wheelchair access. Often, it is the simple, apparently obvious things which are either taken for granted or overlooked. Users themselves are good at ensuring such details are not overlooked, as, for them, they are extremely important.

Be honest about what you are trying to achieve

If all you really want is people to understand or sign up to something that has already been determined, then say so. Do not give people the impression that they will have more influence or involvement than is realistic. Make it clear that we have to work within certain constraints and restrictions (eg. financial, National Service frameworks). It is important not to make assumptions about people's level of knowledge about how your particular service operates. It is embarrassing and even insulting for users to attend events where a level of background or general knowledge, about the question at hand is assumed, but not possessed by individuals taking part.

If you make a commitment to share information, then keep it!

It can be damaging to credibility and future co-operation if this does not happen or if a commitment is reneged upon. Openness and accountability are important facets of the public sector as, of course, is individual patient confidentiality. Be clear about what you can and cannot provide in the way of background material and feedback, and then stick to it.

Start with an open mind

If you attempt to second-guess what people will say or do if you involve them, you negate the point of doing so. If you have already made up your mind on an issue and are engaging people purely as a tick-box exercise, then it is almost certainly going to be a waste of everyone's time and resources. In such circumstances, reading this chapter is also a waste of time!

Consider ethical questions

It can be very demoralising, frustrating, and even costly, to embark upon a model for participation, only to find the results are invalidated because you actually required, for example, approval for the methodology from an ethics committee. Also, bear in mind that strong ethical stances are required in involvement processes, just as they are in service delivery models. There are also peripheral, quasi-ethical questions to consider. Would it be right, for example, to send a middle-aged male manager to discuss intimate issues such as sexual health and teenage pregnancy with a group of teenaged girls?

Make the effect/impact visible

Be prepared to demonstrate what effect or impact participation has had on whatever it is you are actually trying to do. If the answer is 'little or none', then be prepared to justify that, or explain why. Always remember that we are charged with making proper decisions, not necessarily the most popular ones. However, if people have been involved in a number of involvement initiatives and are always or almost always over-ruled, then the purpose and methodology — even the underlying philosophy — could be seriously flawed.

Provide feedback

People expect it and should have a right to it. This is particularly important when feeding back negative information such as why your organisation is not prepared to act upon the views of service users. Honesty, tact, clarity and style are vital considerations here.

It usually takes twice as long and costs twice as much as you think!

Be realistic about the time and resources needed — including the level of expertise. Identify sources of funding and a timetable at the earliest stage possible. If this area of work is new to you or your organisation, consider networking with others who have already been undertaking such work. Most people are quite happy to share best practice information and give advice.

Patients and local people are individuals and, as such, tend to be unpredictable and have different perceptions to our own

Prepare to hear the unexpected and embrace it. Assume nothing and allow differences to be recognised as valid and even valuable. If everyone's opinions were either the same as our own or entirely predictable, there would be no point, whatsoever, in investing time, effort and resources in participation work.

Stay objective throughout the process

It is very damaging if what you say to encourage involvement turns out, by the end of the exercise, to have changed or, worse still, not to have been true in the first place. If the goalposts have to move, make sure people know about it, understand it, and can still play on the same pitch.

Key points

- ✻ Service users now have more opportunities for participation and partnership with professionals, although there are considerable variations in 'the depth and quality of user and public participation'. Service uses have 'a responsibility to be active partners'. Clinical governance involves participation of patients and the public in the NHS. This includes involving them in decisions about acceptable levels of discomfort and risk.

- ✻ Service user and public participation is a major objective of Somerset Health Authority, which set up health panels to involve the public in decision making. Proposals for discussion are invited from organisations concerned with health and local social services. A topic guide is prepared for panel members, who are representative of local communities. Venues have disabled access and facilities. A small payment is made for attendance and any travel costs.

⌘ Meetings are 'always run by an experienced independent facilitator', usually with discussion on two or three topics. Reports, based on the meetings, are made available to local media, sent to panel participants and stakeholders; and debated in a public meeting of Somerset Health Authority.

⌘ A variety of topics has been debated. Independent research found that 'in more than 70% of cases', panel views 'had a direct impact on service planning and/or delivery'. The panels have been widely publicised on local and national media. In a television interview, former members made positive comments about their participation.

⌘ Research found that a majority of general practitioners did not know of the panels' existence or were not convinced of their value. Efforts have been made to address this. A number of 'partner agencies' have started their own panels. These are useful in health service planning.

⌘ The author's guidelines for involving service users include: making initial decisions about the purpose of participation; involving service 'users and the public in planning the participation process itself'; honesty about the amount of participation and its constraints and limits; keeping commitments to share information; having an 'open mind'; considering ethical questions; giving feedback, including explanations about the impact of participation; and being aware of the time involved, likely differences of opinion and need for objectivity.

References

Davidson GW, Seaton MA, Simson J, eds (1989) *Chambers Concise Dictionary*. Chambers, Cambridge
Department of Health (1998) *A First Class Service: Quality in the New NHS*. DoH, London
Department of Health (1999) *Patient and Public Involvement in the New NHS*. DoH, London
Department of Health (2000) *The NHS Plan. A Plan for Investment. A Plan for Reform*. DoH, London
Hogg C (1999) *Patients, Power and Politics: from patients to citizens*. Sage, London

16

Service user and carer participation in colorectal cancer services

Nicky Pearson

Chapter 15 outlined ways in which Somerset Health Authority has developed clinical governance, in partnership with patients and members of local communities, with particular reference to the Somerset health panels. The present chapter describes another clinical governance initiative by Somerset Health Authority: the involvement of patients and their informal carers in the accreditation process for colorectal cancer services. This participation has ensured a high standard of care and treatment.

Related research

Several recent studies have considered the perspectives of individuals with a diagnosis of cancer and/or those of their informal carers. Dougall *et al* (2000) review the extent to which quantitative patient satisfaction surveys adequately assess the needs of patients. These authors outline views expressed in in-depth interviewing with patients with colorectal cancer. Other researchers have studied specific aspects of treatment, including the use of drugs (Redmond, 1998) and needs for palliative care (Osse *et al*, 2000; Young, 2000). Patients' experiences of pain and its treatment have been researched (Maunsell *et al*, 2000), as have the unmet needs of people with cancer (Sanson-Fisher *et al*, 2000) and their quality of life (Chang, 2000; Salander *et al*, 2000). Söllner *et al* (2000) outline research on patient coping, in relation to the use of both traditional and complementary medicine.

The need for patient information, and communication between health professionals and patients and carers has also been explored (Luker *et al*, 2000; Maguire, 2000; Taylor, 2000). Other research has concerned the participation and empowerment of patients who are dying (Martin, 1998; Sahlberg-Blom *et al*, 2000); and the views of people close to individuals who have died while receiving health care (Rogers *et al*, 2000).

The Somerset Health Authority colorectal cancer services study

The aim of this exercise was to gain a deeper understanding of patients' experiences, perceptions and aspirations for cancer services. This is particularly important because positive mental attitude has been shown to correlate with survival advantage in many different types of cancer (Brannon and Feist, 2000; Taylor, 1999). An important aspect of accreditation in cancer services in Somerset concerns patients' satisfaction with the entire process which they experience, throughout their contact with our service. Patient satisfaction is considered to be a key component of service delivery, and this was reflected in the research design.

The study of colorectal cancer services was the second of a series of reviews of patient and carer experience of services covering the main cancer sites. The first site examined was breast cancer and a report is currently being prepared on services for women with gynaecological cancers, after a similar exercise using the same research methods. Plans are now in hand to continue with this exercise and focus on other cancers to coincide with the accreditation process for each.

Ethical issues and research methods

In early 1998, a random sample of patients, stratified by age, sex and year of diagnosis (either 1991/2 or 1995/6) was obtained from pathology results from each of Somerset's two acute NHS Trusts. Prior to any approach to patients, contact was made with their consultants. Patients then received letters from consultants, expressing the latter's support for the study and informing patients that they would be invited to take part. The local research ethics committee also supported the study and patients' GPs were kept fully informed.

During October and November, 1998, a highly regarded independent researcher conducted a series of small focus groups and interviews. A total of forty patients and carers participated. A topic guide was developed to guide discussions through each stage of the illness, diagnosis and treatment, incorporating as many as possible of the standards for the accreditation of colorectal cancer services.

Discussions were taped, transcribed and summarised in report form, and shared with those who took part. This ensured accurate reflection of the key points of the discussions. Summaries were also sent to the accreditation panel for specialist colorectal cancer services for Avon, Somerset and Wiltshire, prior to the team's accreditation visits to local NHS trusts in January 1999. The summaries later became part of the team's overall accreditation report. These focus groups and interviews worked extremely well and raised a number of issues which participants had not previously discussed with anyone. A number of common themes emerged, as well as particular individual experiences highlighting issues of the quality of care received, and patients' experiences and perceptions of cancer services. During the group and individual interviews, some patients expressed the view that the consultation exercise in itself was helpful in dealing with the emotional and psychological aspects of their situation. A number of studies have found that the psychological needs of people with cancer are often unmet (Maguire, 2000; Sanson-Fisher *et al*, 2000); and that support groups effectively enable many of these individuals to share experiences with others in a similar situation (Brannon and Feist, 2000). In the present survey, patients referred to the need for such opportunities. The following are verbatim quotes from participants:

> I don't think about it now, unless I've got a pain — sometimes you do get a pain and you think 'Oh, I wonder if it has come back', and the pain goes next day and you're all right, you know, you just gotta think positive and get on and live on from day-to-day — that's what I think. And it makes you think like that... But it certainly makes a difference being able to talk about it to — I've never met anybody till I came here, to know that they'd had the same thing as I had... And it certainly helps, you know, to think that you've all gone through the same, you know, symptoms.
>
> ... I think this within itself shows there is a need for somebody to get the people together who's had bowel cancer, and be able to talk about it...
>
> Now, if they could say, once a month, have something like this in one of the health centres locally, or in Butleigh Hospital, or in Wells, where a whole group of people that have had the same thing done could get together and say: 'Oh, I get that — ooh, that's like I am!' You know, then you'd think 'Is it' you know, you get a pain – I do now... You know, and I think you could just get a little group of people... That first six months, I have never felt so isolated. I mean I had my family round me and they couldn't have been more supportive if they'd tried.

The main issues discussed in the focus groups and individual interviews were:

- identifying the problem
- referral to hospital
- diagnostic tests
- receiving the diagnosis
- treatment
- before the operation
- after the operation
- relief of symptoms
- monitoring and follow-up
- chemotherapy and radiotherapy
- use of catheters
- transport to outpatient clinics
- support from health service workers
- support from social services
- support from friend, family and neighbours
- stoma care
- complementary therapies
- complaints.

Those who participated made a total of sixteen recommendations for service change. These ranged from relatively straightforward issues to do with the environment of care, such as better privacy and washing facilities in hospitals, to more challenging recommendations: reducing waiting times for referrals to specialists. These recommendations were influential when the accreditation team made its final report and, in some respects, are reflected in the team's recommendations to each NHS trust providing colorectal cancer services for Somerset patients. Other recommendations have been, and continue to be, taken up with individual trusts by the health authority and the Avon, Somerset and Wiltshire Cancer Services Group. In fact, the group followed up all the recommendations made by patients and carers with each trust within six months and, each one has now been implemented.

There seems little doubt that the exercise had a number of highly positive outcomes, including opportunities for patients and carers to communicate. Research suggests that there have often been communication difficulties between health professionals and people with cancer. This is partly because of withdrawal by staff, who fear over-identification with patients' suffering, or are concerned about the psychological impact of openly discussing patients' diagnoses with them (Luker *et al*, 2000; Maguire, 2000; Taylor, 1999). Patients may be reluctant to discuss anxieties because they 'believe that nothing can be done to resolve them. Moreover, they do not want to burden health professionals' (Maguire, 2000, p. 556). In addition, patients may be reluctant to criticise services, even if given the opportunity to do so (Dougall *et al*, 2000).

In contrast, the Somerset Health Authority study enabled several patients and carers to discuss openly issues which, previously, they had kept to themselves – partly because they did not know whom to contact, and partly through a misplaced belief that it would reflect badly on professionals to whom they felt grateful. It also enabled a wealth of information about patients' experiences and perceptions to come through. This has been most helpful in encouraging healthcare teams and individual professionals to reassess the services that they provide from the patients' perspectives. This is extremely important, as without such information, professionals tend to judge services by their own values, which are known to be out of step with patients' concerns (Dougall *et al*, 2000).

Finally, it has had a real and positive impact on the way these services are actually provided, making them more patient centred and patient sensitive. There is considerable evidence to show that patients' satisfaction with the process of care delivery (and prior understanding of what to expect) has a direct positive impact on their response to treatment and, ultimately, on survival rates (Ley, 1995; Taylor, 1999).

Key points

⌘ As part of a clinical governance and accreditation initiative, Somerset Health Authority researched service users' and carers' 'experiences, perceptions and aspirations for cancer services'. Transcripts of discussions were shared with respondents to ensure 'accurate reflection of the key points' discussed.

⌘ As in studies conducted elsewhere, participants commented on the need for support groups. Other issues arising from focus groups and individual interviews concerned referral, diagnosis, treatment, symptom relief, specific treatments, 'monitoring and feedback', transport, support and complaints.

⌘ Participants made 'sixteen recommendations for service change'. These influenced the accreditation team's report to Somerset Health Authority and recommendations to trusts providing relevant services. All the recommendations have been implemented.

⌘ In contrast to findings of other research of professionals' communication difficulties with individuals with cancer, 'the Somerset Health Authority study enabled several patients and carers to openly discuss issues'. The research has also used participants' views to make services 'more patient centred and patient sensitive'. Other studies suggest that patient satisfaction affects treatment response and survival rates.

The publishers and editors acknowledge, with thanks, IBC UK Conferences Limited for copyright permission to publish material previously published in IBC UK Conferences Limited (2000) *Involving Users in Clinical Governance. Working with Users to Provide a Quality Service. LH 183. Conference Handbook for One Day Conference.* 31 March, 2000 at The Marlborough Hotel, London.

References

Brannon L, Feist J (2000) *Health Psychology. An Introduction to Behaviour and Health.* 4th edn. Wadsworth/Thomson Learning, Belmont, CA

Dougall A, Russell A, Rubin G, Ling J (2000) Rethinking patient satisfaction: patient experiences of an open access flexible sigmoidoscopy service. *Soc Sci Med* **5**(1): 53–62

Ley P (1995) Improving patients' understanding, recall, satisfaction and compliance. In: Broome AK, Llewellyn S, eds. 2nd edn. *Health Psychology: Processes and Applications.* Chapman and Hall, London: chap 5

Luker KA, Austin L, Caress A, Hallett CE (2000) The importance of 'knowing the patient': community nurses' constructions of quality in providing palliative care. *J Adv Nurs* **31**(4): 775–82

Maguire P (2000) Managing psychological morbidity in cancer patients. *Eur J Cancer* **36**(5): 556–8

Martin GW (1998) Empowerment of dying patients: the strategies and barriers to patient autonomy. *J Adv Nurs* **28**(4): 737–44

Maunsell E, Allard P, Dorval M, Labbé J (2000) A brief pain diary for ambulatory patients with advanced cancer. Acceptability and validity. *Cancer* **88**(10): 2387–97

Osse BHP, Vernooij-Danssen J, de Vree BPW, Schadé E, Grol RPTH (2000) Assessment of the need for palliative care as perceived by individual cancer patients and their families. *Cancer* **88**(4): 900–11

Ramsey SD, Andersen MR, Etzioni R, Moinpour C, Peacock S, Potosky A, Urban N (2000) Quality of life in survivors of colorectal carcinoma. *Cancer* **88**(6): 1294–1303

Redmond K (1998) Assessing patients' needs and preferences in the management of advanced colorectal cancer. *Br J Cancer* **77** Supplement 2: 5–7

Rogers A, Karlsen S, Addington-Hall J (2000) 'All the services were excellent. it is when the human element comes in that things go wrong': Dissatisfaction with hospital care in the last year of life. *J Adv Nurs* **31**(4): 768–74

Sahlberg-Blom E, Ternestadt BM, Johansson JE (2000) Patient participation in decision making at the end of life as seen by a close relative. *Nurs Ethics* **7**(4): 296–311

Salander P, Bergenheim AT, Henriksson R (2000) How was life after treatment of a malignant brain tumour? *Soc Sci Med* **51**(4): 589–98

Sanson-Fisher R, Girgis A, Boyes A, Bonevski B, Burton L, Cook P (2000) The unmet supportive care needs of patients with cancer. *Cancer* **88**(1): 226–37

Söllner W, Maislinger S, DeVries A, Steixner E, Rumpold G, Lukas P (2000) Use of complementary and alternative medicine by cancer patients is not associated with perceived distress or poor compliance with standard treatment but with active coping behaviour. *Cancer* **89**(4): 873–80

Taylor S (1999) *Health Psychology.* 4th edn. McGraw Hill, Boston

Young C (2000) Palliative care in Korea: a nursing point of view. *Progress in Palliative Care* **8**(1): 12–16

17

Self-help: personal perspectives and experiences

Andrew Wetherell and Roberta Graley-Wetherell

Andrew Wetherell

I first became aware of the amazing power of self-help support when I was receiving in-patient treatment for depression back in the early part of 1994. This followed an eight-month struggle with the illness, which culminated with the loss of my job in December, 1993.

Anyone who has a first-hand experience of the nightmare scenario of depression and anxiety will be well-aware of just how awful it feels and how an individual can feel totally isolated and devoid of hope. Shortly following admission for treatment, and having met a number of other service users who all had various types of depression, I was astonished to learn that there were other people like me — people who understood what I was going through, who accepted me and who offered me unconditional support, respect and empathy.

A highly significant factor in the self-help process is the mutual benefit experienced by everyone involved. It appears to me that all too often we see or experience one-way experiences in life, and to be part of something which is broadly of mutual benefit to all participants has to be a worthwhile and highly positive use of time.

While the care and treatment I received during my stay as an in-patient was of high quality and of great assistance to me, I would have to say that the largest single factor of most benefit was meeting other people who could empathise with what I was experiencing. All too often during my illness, I was given the useless advice of 'pull yourself together' by a selection of colleagues and friends — something which the group of people I met during my in-patient admission would never have said because they knew it was one of the worst things that you can say to someone in that situation.

While one door shut firmly behind me following the loss of my job, a whole array of other opportunities opened up as I recovered from my depression. In the spring of 1994, and fuelled by the enlightening experience of meeting other people with similar problems to my own, I spent the next two years working on a voluntary unpaid basis setting up and running self-help support groups in my home town.

In conjunction with someone I met while receiving treatment, I set up and ran a self-help support group for people with the broad range of mental health problems. Having received so much from others in my own personal journey, I started off and continued with the philosophy of 'perhaps I can help just one other person'. Knowing how devastating mental health problems can be, I just wanted to share my experience and hopefully assist others in dealing with their problems.

Pleasingly, I have learnt that the group I founded has helped a number of people — not just the one I had originally hoped for, and this is, of course, a wonderful reward and most reassuring. It also has to be said that while I was engaging in the voluntary work, I was helping myself as well. It gave me a purpose in life, something to focus on, a structure to my day and assisted me greatly in building up my self-worth and confidence. Ultimately, it led to a new and far more enjoyable and rewarding career in the mental health world, for which I am grateful.

The general mental health self-help support group which I founded and ran, led me to help facilitate a more specialist group for people with obsessive compulsive disorder and associated illnesses. Again, this was a most positive experience for me and the group helped a large number of people to help themselves through the sharing of experiences, unconditional acceptance, support and empathy, all of which took place in a mutually beneficial way.

As far as self-help is concerned, for me the philosophy behind it is akin to the proverb about if you give someone a fish, you feed them for a day, but if you teach them to fish, they will be able to feed themselves for a lifetime (Oxfam), simple but largely true.

Another observation I have in relation to self-help support is how universal it is. It does not matter if the subject area is mental health, cancer, bereavement, victims of crime, etc., the core values and principles hold true and are equally valid across the spectrum. I guess this also means, generally, that there really should not be any need these days for anyone to be isolated, struggling on their own and having no one to turn to.

However, one of the problems facing self-help initiatives is the issue of funding and there are so many good groups grinding to a halt just because they cannot pay their rent to meet up once a week. Sadly, it seems to me that there are still health, social services departments and other organisations who just do not understand how powerful and cost-effective self-help can be. It is the old saying about some people know the cost of everything and the value of nothing — this is a culture we need to get away from and education of the powers that be may have an important role to play.

Probably one of the best examples that exists of self-help is, of course, Alcoholics Anonymous (AA), which must be the biggest and most successful self-help organisation in existence. I think it is wonderful that wherever you may happen to be in the world, the chance is that there will be an AA group meeting within reasonable access! Their tried and tested twelve-step approach has also been adapted for other uses, such as drug use and gambling, proving the massive value and universal application of self-help.

Below, I have listed just a few pointers/key issues which I found of assistance when running a self-help support group.

A structured approach is usually helpful, so there would be a start and finish time together with some basic ground rules, such as:

❖ No racist, ageist, sexist or abusive remarks.

❖ Only one person talking at a time.

❖ Respect others in the same way you expect to receive respect.

❖ No one should be pressurised to speak, but the facilitator(s) will actively encourage and support full participation of everyone.

❖ Confidentiality — The AA Yellow Card approach of 'Who you see here, what you hear here, when you leave here, let it stay here' is a sound one.

❖ Let the facilitator(s) know if there is any way the sessions can be improved.

❖ Good facilitation is essential — **and an art**! There is a need to assist quieter people to speak when they want to and also to know when and how to stop someone who is unfairly monopolising the session to the detriment of others.

❖ No giving of advice! The focus has to be on the sharing of experiences and of mutual empathy.

❖ It is important to exchange contact details with others within the group, as appropriate, in order that people have access to mutual support and understanding between meetings.

❖ It can be helpful to engage in social activities together outside of the group setting.

❖ All participants need to be encouraged to have an ownership of the group. For example, one person might bring the milk and sugar, another the tea, and so on.

There can be quite a bond which develops between people who come together with a common problem in a mutual self-help support forum.

One key issue of concern is how easy it can be for a highly motivated and enthusiastic person to get 'burnt-out' while running a self-help group. As with most activities (eg. the local tennis club) a great amount can be left to one or two main individuals. This, I believe, needs to be avoided as far as possible, with the various tasks within the group being shared. This not only leads to reduced pressures on the one or two naturally active individuals, but it also assists all participants to have that ownership of the group mentioned above.

Roberta Graley-Wetherell

It was way back in 1982, when I decided that maybe what I needed was help of a different sort. I had been experiencing mental health problems since I was sixteen — now I was twenty-seven and not much further down the path of recovery than when I first sought help from the statutory psychiatric services. I was on my eighth admission to the local psychiatric hospital and repeating the same pattern yet again, mental distress followed by 'self-medication' (taking the form of excessive drinking and drug abuse), which again would lead to even more mental distress. I needed to break the cycle so I decided to go to a self-help group. Unfortunately, there was not a lot around at the time, so I went to AA — at least I could address part of my problem.

What I did find was a lot of support and empathy and, more importantly, I felt I was not judged. I was not made to feel that I was a weak or lesser person because of my problems. I was with people who really understood that sometimes reality can be so painful and intolerable that the only way to survive is to escape — even if it is only for a short while. What I was also forced to face was that until I really addressed what was happening to me and why, then no matter how stoned I got, it would still be there when I eventually came back to reality. Talking with these people who had similar experiences gave me the strength to start on my road back to a tolerable reality. I gained so much knowledge from these new friends that I learnt how to manage my distress better, to recognise that there were certain situations that triggered my anxiety and that these were to be avoided whenever possible — or I needed to keep a degree of control over them. I not only learnt my coping strategies from the group but also, by seeing how members had climbed back from depths greater than I had reached, gave me the confidence to start my own climb back. Having such good role models, who were there at the end of the telephone for me whenever I needed extra support, was invaluable.

I knew this was not the only model and decided that maybe others would benefit from the simple, open and honest forum of shared experiences. To this end, I set up a group for anyone who had a drug problem or who was affected by drugs in their lives. It was attended by recovering addicts, carers, friends and families of addicts and occasionally, addicts who were still using drugs (usually going through a withdrawal programme). This for me, was quite an exciting part of my life. I was taking the initiative to develop a group which might lessen others' distress, and this was probably the first time since I was a child that I was doing something I felt really positive about. The group was quite successful and eventually, I moved on but the group continued — its natural progression was that it developed into a relatives, friends and carers' group. Later with a friend, I set up a Narcotics Anonymous group. This was around 1984 and, much to my delight, I heard recently that the group is still running and has helped hundreds of addicts in my home city.

I was very much involved with other projects as well as the 'Twelve Stepping Groups'. During my spare time, I enjoyed doing voluntary work and some of this work brought me into contact with self-help groups of all kinds. I spent six weeks of one summer working on a school holiday's play scheme for families with children who had disabilities. The scheme was set up and run by a self-help group called 'Smile Don't Stare!'. The group was for parents and families with children who had severe learning difficulties, physical disabilities and terminal illness. The parents had had negative experiences trying to get their children onto regular summer play schemes.

They found when attending the group that many of them were dreading the long summer break when schools closed for six or seven weeks, for while their able-bodied children were welcome to join the local community schemes, the children with disabilities were not allowed to join them. This caused parental exhaustion, and unnecessary conflict.

The group managed to secure some funding from the local authorities and a youth club allowed them to use their premises during the day free of charge. They then recruited volunteers to help out. These were not just friends and relatives but students who were on their summer break. They arranged activities and games for the children and a day trip to a theme park, zoo or such like once a week. The most rewarding part of the scheme was that all the family could join in and the children made new friends. In particular, the ones who were able bodied could share the problems they had living with a sibling who had severe disabilities. Self-help for kids! We often overlook the fact that children living in families with these problems also need support. It certainly taught me a lot about all kinds of disabilities and about carers' needs. It was also one of the best summers I have ever had — I really enjoyed myself.

During this time, I had also got involved with self-help of a different kind. The kind which is about self-advocacy, patients' rights and campaigning. The psychiatric services were still playing a big part in my life and although my days of drug abuse were behind me, I was still having regular treatment for depression and anxiety problems and other residual problems from my youth like eating disorders and self-harm. Although the services were doing all they could, I felt they were doing it to me rather than its being of **my** choosing. I decided that I wanted to do all I could to change the system so that it met more effectively the needs of people like myself. I joined the newly formed Patients' Council which was the first in the United Kingdom. This was exciting and ground-breaking work and we were all bonded by a common cause. I am lucky enough to still have some of those people in my life and they are still the people I turn to when I need support.

It was around this time that I moved to another town. I gave up my 'normal' job and decided to devote my time to the development of what is often called the mental health service user movement. I set up and facilitated groups in the town I had moved to and the local psychiatric services were extremely supportive of these initiatives. The local social services allowed us to open the day centre at the weekends and have it as a service user-run drop in. We had a social group for people who found it hard to mix and also arranged theatre trips, visited art galleries, had days at the coast or simply an evening at the local pub.

I also set up a Patients' Council in the local acute unit which could raise issues which affected many or all of the patients. In addition, I managed to obtain funding for a local telephone help-line.

This was initially for people who were in emotional distress, and wanted to speak to someone out of normal statutory services hours or who did not want to access statutory services for whatever reason (often because of the stigma associated with mental illness). It was through this work that I identified another need which was not being met in my local area.

The small rural town I had moved to was friendly but could also be quite judgemental and sadly, people were not very well informed about certain things like mental health and HIV/Aids issues. I had to go into the local hospital for a routine operation and I had already had my pre-med. I was waiting to be taken down to theatre when one of the doctors noticed on my notes that I had a history of drug abuse. He then came to see me and in a very loud voice on an open ward, demanded to know if I had been tested for HIV recently and, if not, he said that they must do it now to ensure his staff were not infected as I was a high-risk patient. I was extremely distraught and I agreed to the blood test. The doctor who appeared in gown, mask and gloves took a sample of blood but managed to spray it up the side of my locker and part of the wall. This threw everyone into a panic.

A nurse appeared a few minutes later in similar attire but holding a bottle of bleach and a jay cloth! She scrubbed and cleaned and eventually I went to theatre. I was discharged as soon as I could stand on my own and they even paid for the taxi home. It felt like they could not get rid of me quick enough but I did not complain, I just wanted to get out of there, as soon as I physically could.

The whole experience left me traumatised and I needed to talk about it. I could not find anything in the local self-help directory and ended up telling my therapist. He was appalled and put in an official complaint. I heard nothing for several weeks, then, out of the blue, came a call from the Aids Liaison Officer who left a message for me at the local MIND office, where I worked in a voluntary capacity. I was frantic when I got the message to call her and a colleague sat with me for an hour or so discussing all the possibilities. I naturally thought that they were calling about my blood test and I, of course, feared the worst — even though I did not know of anyone who I had shared needles with having been diagnosed HIV positive, there was always a chance. Eventually, with my colleague holding my hand, I rang her back. She did not know anything about my test and had only called to ask if I would be willing to help her set up a self-help support group in the area for people living with HIV and AIDS.

When she heard my story, she was absolutely livid and supported my complaint. Eventually, I got an apology from the local hospital and I decided that I would approach them for funding to set up telephone information and a help line for the area. Using the 'carrot and stick' approach, we explained that it would be much to their credit if they set up such a service in a rural area (it was only 1989 and there were very few areas with such a provision). Further, I promised that I would not sue or go to the press with my story if they did this. We got the funding. In 1990, we managed to run a training programme facilitated by trainers from the National Aids Line and we were up and running by the end of the year. We managed to allay many people's fears, persuade people who were at risk to get proper medical testing — with pre- and post-test counselling — and to make quality information available throughout the region.

All throughout this period, I was still working in the mental health service user movement and had now managed not only to be participating in services at a local level, but also nationally. Locally, I was part of several planning and strategy groups and nationally I had joined the Department of Health on their Mental Health Task Force. This for me was a great achievement because at last I was not only participating in the changing and improvement of local services, but also influencing Government policy.

In 1992, I was invited to a conference in Holland to explore the possibilities of setting up a European Network of Mental Health Service Users — it was amazing! Over sixty service users came from twenty-six countries. All had such varied and differing experiences and yet they all shared a common experience of being totally disempowered by the services which were supposed to be there to help them. I joined the steering group and became a member of the committee and eventually, was voted in as the Founder Chairperson in 1994. It felt quite far removed from the experiences I had had as a sixteen-year-old in total distress, with no-one to share it with. Now I had friends all over the world who understood; did not judge and totally supported me. Seeing colleagues from Eastern Europe who had struggled to get there and were fascinated by the food available in the hotel restaurant made me realise just how important it is to offer support to our peers. We were all there because of a common experience, an experience we felt others would not completely understand unless they themselves had been through it — the common experience of having a mental health problem which is often labelled as abnormal, unacceptable and leaves people being stigmatised by the rest of their community. The social issues of our respective countries and our cultures were swept aside and we became bonded in a common experience.

While I was the Chairperson of the European Network, I was asked to go to several European Parliament advisory groups about disabilities. It was at one of these meetings that I met Terry. He was heavily involved with a peer support/self-help/campaigning organisation called the UK Coalition of People Living with HIV and AIDS. Terry was extremely interested in my work back home in the field of peer advocacy. I had been working for the United Kingdom Advocacy Network — a national umbrella group of advocacy projects, service user forums and self-help groups who are involved in planning, informing or trying to change the service they use. Importantly, all of their affiliated groups are specifically run by and for people who have experienced emotional distress/mental ill-health.

When we returned to England, I travelled to London to meet up with Terry and some of his colleagues. We put in a funding proposal for a peer advocacy project in Kensington, Chelsea and Westminster, a London Borough with a high population of people living with HIV or AIDS. It was accepted and we advertised for volunteers and then ran a training programme delivered by myself and the project co-ordinator. We based the project on peer advocacy in mental health but we adapted the training to meet the needs of people living with HIV or Aids. It was most successful and eventually the service was extended to Manchester and now is growing still. An example of how self-help groups can learn from each other.

I now, jointly with my husband, Andrew, run a commercial mental health consultancy. We do lots of training, service development, research and evaluations. We work mainly in mental health but we are happy to take on work from other areas as well and this is thanks to the confidence, knowledge and skills that I feel I have built up during my time in self-help. Unfortunately, we have to work on a commercial basis because we have to pay our bills and put a roof over our heads. Self-help groups are usually free to attend, unless they ask for a small donation towards running costs. All the hours spent supporting each other are given for free, the administration and facilitation is again often on a voluntary basis. It is an area which attracts very little funding and yet no-one denies that the services provided by self-help groups are often much more effective in the long-term than statutory services. Therefore, I plead with anyone reading this who has the power to allocate budgets not to forget how cost-effective self-help support groups can be. Please spare a little of those precious funds to bridge a gap often identified by service users, but all too rarely addressed by service commissioners.

Key points

❡ Inspired by their own experiences, the authors have been involved in setting up and running many diverse self-help groups, and self-help concerned with 'self-advocacy, patients' rights and campaigning'. The establishment of patients' councils, and a mental health consultancy are also outlined. One of the authors was determined to change her experience of services being 'done to' her.

❡ Self-help is of universal value in relation to a wide range of health care and other needs. Key issues in the running of self-help groups include: establishing structure; respect for others; avoidance of discriminatory remarks; enabling individuals to talk without feeling pressured or talked over; ensuring confidentiality; avoidance of advice; availability of members' contact details; and shared membership of, and responsibility in, the group.

❡ Benefits of self-help groups include: empowerment from participation; individuals' realisation that they are not alone with their problems; acceptance, support and empathy; sharing experiences; learning positive coping strategies; and the availability of positive role models.

❡ In one self-help group, parents of children with disabilities and terminal illnesses secured funding for activities for these children, with involvement of whole families and volunteers. One benefit was the opportunity for non-disabled siblings to share their problems.

❡ One of the authors experienced considerable stigmatisation and insensitivity from professionals in relation to assumed HIV positive status. This inspired her to establish, with funding, a local telephone line concerned with HIV/AIDS, a training programme and a peer advocacy group in this area.

❡ The European Network of Mental Health Service Users has members in twenty-six countries, who have all experienced considerable disempowerment in services. One of the authors has been founding Chair of this organisation. She has also been involved in 'service planning and strategy groups' and in the Department of Health Mental Health Task Force, influencing Central Government policy.

❡ It is sometimes difficult to obtain adequate funding for self-help groups, despite their cost effectiveness.

18

The good, the bad and the ugly: the role of local radio as a medium for overcoming prejudice

Roger Phillips

Introduction

There is evidence that stigmatisation can be disempowering for both health service users and their carers (Oliver and Barnes, 1998; Pilgrim and Waldron, 1998; Sayce, 2000). These individuals, as well as staff and hospital management, can experience stigmatisation as a result of adverse press publicity. When investigative journalism is unchecked by ethical and moral consideration, the resulting covert and intrusive techniques may play a significant part in the perpetuation of stigma, and may reduce morale for those associated with the 'story'.

Conversely, the general public and media professionals may feel disempowered if they do not receive the information to which they consider they are entitled.

In a society with reasonable freedom of information, the users of any health service include members of the public, who have an interest in and a right to know what goes on within its walls. Improvements in some hospitals appear to have occurred, at least in part, because of investigative journalism into unsatisfactory and sometimes appalling conditions. In some cases, journalists' reports have stimulated Government inquiries, and subsequent reforms that have benefited service users. In addition, journalists have reported on positive innovations or been at the forefront of campaigns that express pride in their local services and may be seen as empowering. An early example is the account by Charles Dickens and WH Wills of the work of St Lukes' 'Hospital for the Insane' and the patients' Christmas celebrations at this institution. This account, originally published in *Household Words* in 1852, was used by the hospital as a promotional pamphlet (Stone, 1969, p. 381), a pioneering example of a health service working proactively with the media.

In the past, some aspects of health care, particularly mental health, have been practised away from the public gaze and have not been accountable. Transparency is a key word in providing services which meet the public's demand for accountable care, and the media, in this case local radio, has an important role to play in providing information and an objective enlightenment for the public.

One of the great newspaper magnates of the past, Lord Northcliffe, said that journalism is 'a profession whose business it is to explain to others what it personally does not understand', and there is no doubt that, as a presenter working for the BBC in Liverpool, Radio Merseyside, I lack any of the qualifications with which the other contributors to this book are so eminently endowed.

Merseyside is where Ashworth Special Hospital (a high security hospital) is cited, and it is inevitable that the subject of mental health and offenders surfaces from time to time as a topic for discussion on the daily phone-in which I present. Callers range from staff to former offenders and victims — and, of course, the general public, whose knowledge of mental health and Ashworth is, to put it politely, fairly limited. I do have a particular view of the way Ashworth operates with the media, and the way that both the media and the public view Ashworth.

The author's perceptions are separated into three sections:

1. The past: The 'bad old days' and what can be learnt from what was wrong with those bad old days, as seen from my side of the microphone.
2. The present: The 'good, the bad and the ugly', the changes slowly getting underway.
3. The future: 'for better or worse' — some suggestions as to where to aim for.

Why local radio?

First, though, a few words about why you should be bothered about local radio at all — apart from the fact that it keeps me in a job! There are two main reasons:

❖ It's a good route to national coverage. The BBC used to be terrible at communicating with itself, but modern technology and a different culture, have led to much more interaction. And so, a story at a local radio station is very often the first route to national coverage. Local radio is the eyes and ears of the Beeb.

But more importantly:

❖ It's the best route to the local community and your staff. Ashworth is an important part of Liverpool and Merseyside. Fifteen hundred or so staff mean that perhaps 5,000 or more people locally have a direct stake in the hospital; and to a greater or lesser extent, this will be true of any hospital, including special hospitals or secure units anywhere in the country. Many patients at Ashworth come from within our local broadcasting area, their relatives are also among our listeners, so too, perhaps, are their victims or victims' relatives. Not least, those people who live around any institution — a school, a nightclub or a special hospital — have an interest in, and a right to know, what goes on within its walls.

Furthermore, the local media can help to engender pride, rather than embarrassment: there are some who work at Ashworth who pretend that they work elsewhere. But it is only with a sense of pride that the psychiatrists, psychologists, nurses, healthcare assistants, cleaners, cooks and security staff will gain the confidence to grow a hospital into the caring community it should be.

Local radio is an excellent way of reaching all those people. In Liverpool, BBC Radio Merseyside has far more listeners than any other speech-based broadcasting station, local or national; it is only on local radio that you will reach all the sections of the local community. It is a medium worth cultivating to help create caring communities both within and outside hospital and other health institutions.

The kind of programme which I present, a phone-in, is important in that cultivation. Every week, I field about one hundred calls on every possible subject, and inevitably, in Liverpool, there are, from time to time, calls about Ashworth, usually when it is in the news, and the calls will usually be along the lines of, 'the patients are all criminals they are mad and bad, they live a life of luxury or they are a waste of money'. Most often, calls come after an inquiry report, of which Ashworth has had several in recent times, concentrating on criticism of staff and management. More often than not, a former patient, a member of staff or a relative of either, will ring in to respond. Sometimes issues arise that need an authoritative reply from the hospital itself, which brings me to the first part of my thesis.

The past: the bad old days

Ashworth was originally two separate hospitals, Park Lane and Moss Side, which merged into Ashworth in 1989 — and they didn't just respond to media enquiries. The stories that got around may or may not have been true, and sadly, many of them were, but, in any event, they were believed and, indeed, have been reinforced by two major inquiries in the nineties: the Blom-Cooper and some seven years later, the Fallon reports. The myths are, to be fair, pretty confused.

On the one hand, a Victorian, Dickensian prison, full of evil criminals contained for the safety of us outside, and (in the past) only the valiant knights of the prison officers association (who were, and still to some extent are, a lot cannier at using the media than management) to keep the lid on the cauldron.

On the other hand, a five-star hotel where so-called psychologists and psychiatrists molly-coddle these disgusting inhuman individuals, who are able to fool the so-called 'professionals' into releasing them back into the community to commit further terrible offences.

If management in the bad old days were aware of the public perceptions, they either did not care or did not know what to do about it. If there was a press or public relations officer, nobody was letting the press or public know. Calls we put in were mainly unanswered — and if they were, no-one was available. The only people who were usually as keen as mustard to talk to us (the media) were the prison officers association. And do not just take my word for it — let me quote from one of the inquiries I just referred to.

Paragraph Section 1.18 of Volume 1 of the Fallon Report looks briefly at the history of the Special Hospitals. Paragraph 10 speaks about management failure by the late '80s, 'the end result was a management vacuum at the local level, a vacuum which the Prison Officers Association "in particular" was happy to fill' (DoH, 1999).

Now, believe it or not, journalists are actually ordinary human beings, and when they meet up with a blank wall, they tend to assume the worst — assume a cover-up (only the guilty have something to hide), and the field is wide open for anyone with a particular axe to grind to feed journalists' and, thereby, the public's imagination, with their prejudices.

The fact is that there have been things to hide at both Park Lane and Moss Side, and subsequently at Ashworth, and I guess that the problems we faced as local media were just another symptom of the bad management that allowed what happened there to develop.

It is great, from the media's point of view, that it was a television documentary programme, *Cutting Edge*, that uncovered some of the wrongdoings that led to the 1992 Blom-Cooper inquiry (Blom-Cooper *et al*, 1992); but that it should be so, is a dreadful indictment of the management of special hospitals at that time and of the Mental Health Act Commission, who were supposed to be overseeing the special hospitals. And, what lessons were learnt? None it appears, in that the subsequent Fallon inquiry, which was called for in February 1997, and reported two years later, was triggered by a patient, who felt his only whistleblowing route was via the media.

To be fair, Ashworth, had by then learned something about dealing with their public image — and one of the senior staff did speak to the media about what had happened — although, by the time he did, it was really far too late and it was, of course, RE-active, rather than PRO-active. News management — and that is really what I am suggesting — is one way to help restore confidence in the community both within and without the walls. But it has to be an on-going, long-term policy, which means that if, or to be realistic when, the next crisis — the next horror story — surfaces, you are able to control the story to minimise the public relations damage.

I know it is difficult — certainly at Ashworth, and undoubtedly elsewhere, because:

- there are many people with axes to grind
- there are undoubtedly things going on of which management are not, I am sure, proud
- there is good work going on, which the less enlightened members of the public and media might well object to.

But things are moving on, and there have been major changes towards an honesty and openness that would have been unthinkable in the bad old days. What is it like now? How honest is honest? How open is open? Is the picture really as I have entitled the second part of my thesis.

The good, the bad and the ugly?

Well, of course it is not. There has been an uphill struggle to change the perceptions of the hospital, both internally and externally. At Ashworth, the decision to change the name was a start — and it **was** important, because it was trying to say to the staff and public that the old culture was being abandoned for a new future. From the media's point of view, it was the appointment of a press and public relations officer that had the most immediate impact. Suddenly, we had someone we could contact to ask questions, someone who was keen to find out our requirements and to build a relationship with the station. Inevitably, that meant someone who wanted to put the best possible gloss on every story — but that is the name of the PR game.

There are two important points here:

❖ The best press officer in the world cannot do the business unless he or she has good and immediate access to very senior management, and are trusted to speak for the organisation themselves.

❖ We don't want to be interviewing press officers — we want to be talking to the people directly involved, the ones making or implementing the decisions.

What is so much better about Ashworth is that that's exactly what we can do: we get a relatively quick response to requests for statements on any issue and, if needed, we get the interviews from the people to whom we want to talk, if at all possible. For example, a chief executive has spoken on our airwaves on more than one occasion about apparent security lapses. In my view, the very fact that people will face up to the questions begins to change the image of the place in both the public's and the staff's minds.

As I mentioned earlier, it is all very well being RE-active — one of the vital functions of the press office, in my view, is to be PRO-active — and, again, Ashworth has been, in fits and starts, improving in that direction. There **are** good news stories to be told to help move the image from that of a prison to that of a therapeutic hospital. Let me give you a couple of examples.

The first is, in a way, the reason I'm writing this today. Some years ago, the then general manager, happened to hear me responding to a critical call about Ashworth — and whatever it was I said in reply to the caller, it encouraged her to invite me to take a look round the place. It was the first such invitation I had had in seventeen years broadcasting within Merseyside — a fact which itself speaks volumes about the past; but an invitation which showed the positive changes that were going on. I had a fascinating day and, of course, I was shown the 'good side' of the hospital; but I was impressed by the way I was allowed to talk to staff and patients who were unhappy about the way the place was run and about the post Blom-Cooper

Inquiry changes. Simply as a result of that visit, I became much better informed to be able to deal with the subject whenever it comes up on a phone-in.

One ward I visited, the high dependency women's ward, seemed to me to be the subject of a possible radio fly-on-the-wall documentary. The sky did not fall apart when I suggested that we would like to make such a programme — and, indeed, we **did** make and broadcast a documentary called *Taking Out the Stitches*. I will explain later some of the difficulties we laboured under in making the programme, but the end result was that, for once, the Merseyside public got some insight into what was happening at Ashworth; Ashworth itself got a better image than it normally does; and we got a good programme out of it at the BBC.

The other PRO-active example around that time was an art exhibition in Liverpool City Centre of work created by some of the patients. Ashworth could not have been more helpful in arranging interviews, giving us access and so on, and again, there was good coverage and a positive image portrayed.

But the truth is that to get the trust of the public, it seems to me that you have to tell the whole story, the good, the bad and the ugly. Ashworth did, at one time, get pretty good at being pro-active when telling the good, although between the revelation of the events which led to the Fallon inquiry, and the inquiry itself , hiding the bad and the ugly got in the way of telling anything in a pro-active way, let alone the good; that was not just with the media, but with civil servants and ministers as well!

Ashworth has, in the past, never been very good at dealing with the media when it comes to the bad and the ugly, although since the Fallon report, it has improved beyond recognition. I remember some three or four years ago, there were a couple of separate rooftop protests. Nobody contacted us from the hospital. There appeared to be various reasons for that, including the idea that because it is a secure hospital, nobody is ever going to know, and that if it were known, it would reflect badly on the place. But very little remains secret from the outside — and we were, of course, tipped off.

If that had happened ten years ago, if we had actually managed to speak to anyone in authority, it would have been a case of 'no comment' or The Official Secrets Act and all that rubbish; what got better is that we do want — and did at that time get — an acknowledgement of what was going on.

The trouble is that we want more than that, and details about the rooftop incidents were conspicuous by their absence. We sent out our radio car, but rather than trying to accommodate our needs, our reporter was asked to leave and threatened with being escorted off the premises if he didn't. There is another way to deal with an incident like that, which will satisfy the needs of both the media and public, and put the hospital in a positive light. As it is, the kind of defensive press relations I have described **can** lead to a very negative image being put across.

Take, for example, a hostage taking incident on one of the wards in June 1994. The internal investigation was seized upon by the staff unions to allege a cover up. Now, I do not know the details of that incident, nor the legal constraints on management, but a reluctance to give details, generalisations such as — and I am quoting here — 'inconsistencies on this particular ward' and 'steps will be taken' and 'redefine philosophy and management', give an impression that there is something going on that is being hidden.

Indeed, the Fallon report bears that out but, importantly, goes on to say: 'had this report (into the ward hostage-taking) been published in 1994, the necessary in-depth examination of the personality disorder unit at Ashworth Hospital would have taken place some years earlier than our inquiry' (DoH, 1999, p. 1). My point is that lack of courage — or common sense — of management to publish, allowed others to take the initiative and lead the agenda in **their** own interests — allegations of mismanagement, stories of an illegal drugs culture throughout the hospital. To be fair to management, they **did** respond to the allegations, but only after we had pushed and pushed for a response and, ultimately, explained that we would run the story one-sided, if no response was forthcoming. I do not know if that problem was over-caution on the press officer's part, she may have just been acting as a buffer between ourselves and 'over-cautious' management, but instances like that put a real strain on the relationship between press officers and the media.

Ashworth and all health institutions including those caring for offenders need to take the initiative. Not just with the good, but with the bad and ugly as well — and that must include what the general public perceives as being bad.

The 1999 White House Conference on Mental Health called for a national anti-stigma campaign. As Donna E Shalala, Secretary of Health and Human Services, said in introducing the report, fear and stigma persist, resulting in lost opportunities for individuals to seek treatment and improve or recover. One of my searching questions relates to why stigma is still so strong? The answer appears to be fear of violence: people with mental illness, especially those with psychosis, are perceived to be more violent than in the past (Collins, 1999). Now the truth is that there is little risk of violence or harm to a stranger from casual contact with an individual who has a mental disorder. So, why is fear of violence so entrenched?

Most research focuses on media coverage and deinstitutionalisation. And yet, many people thought that deinstitutionalisation, which took place in the States as it did in the UK, would reduce stigma as community care and commonplace exposure developed. However, one series of surveys (Angermeyer and Matschinger, 1996) found that selective media reporting reinforced the public's stereotypes, linking violence and mental illness and encouraged people to distance themselves from those with mental disorders. This is a major factor in stigmatisation, and I believe what is true of the United States in this respect is just as true here. How mental health professionals should deal with that, is where I finally turn to now.

For better or worse

There's been a grand tradition of horror stories — real and supposed — about Ashworth: take a genuine headline under the tag 'exclusive' in the *Sunday Mirror*, about a leave of absence trip from Ashworth to the Alton Towers theme park:

Psycho Towers

Three mad killers and a child molester mix with theme park kids

There is talk in the article of a 'depraved sex monster'. I want to answer two questions about that kind of story.

Firstly, why are they there at all? Well, newspaper editors think they sell papers — and they may be right for all I know — but that does not mean that they inevitably have to have the shock horror spin put on them.

Secondly, someone gives them the story. Why? I suppose it has to be one of three reasons, or a combination of them:

1. Financial gain.
2. Someone, presumably in the case I quote, a staff member at Ashworth, has a grievance against management.

3.   Someone disagrees with the rehabilitative aim of such visits.

Let's take the third, first. Although I think it is the least likely reason: if it's a genuine belief by the leaker that such visits are morally wrong, management **can** do something — continuous staff education about all hospital matters, including such outside visits, which are, after all, a proper part of therapy.

You will never stop such stories, you may think, if it is the first two reasons: the leaker is after money or trying to embarrass the hospital, or to dislodge a particular member of staff.

Well, I don't agree with that proposition: it is interesting to note that a subsequent story in another national newspaper, the *Sunday Express*, concerning a patient getting lost on a similar trip elsewhere, got little or no follow-up by the rest of the media, certainly not locally. Why not? I think it is because of changes that were in process at that time: the media were beginning to realise that just because a story concerns Ashworth, it doesn't automatically make it a story. And it was realising that, because the hospital was becoming pro-active — inviting journalists on a one-to-one basis to spend a day looking around the hospital, so that, at least, they could have no misconceptions, as they undoubtedly had in the past. Of course, had there been a genuine escape from the trip, or an attack on a child at Alton Towers, then undoubtedly that would have been a lead story which all the media would have homed in on — and rightly so.

There is an approach which might avoid these kinds of stories and at the same time help to educate the public more widely; a way which might ultimately help in creating caring communities — or at least better informed communities: the starting point of caring. And that is to become pro-active and to try to defuse the tabloid stories. You could go even further.

For example, leave of absence visits are not only defensible, they are an important part of patient care. Why not go on the offensive and argue the case? Maybe, even consider getting consent from the patients and invite the media to cover the trips. I have no idea how many such visits there are, but I am sure that every hospital or unit will know the ones that will get nurse X or administrator Y to tip off his/her favourite journalist. Get in there first — have the courage of your convictions — do not wait for it to get into the public domain outside your control. Educate the staff and educate the public — and improve the chances of caring communities within and without the system.

Doing it through the local media might be the best place to start. You have a big advantage in dealing with your local media, in that we need you as much as you need us. National journalists from radio, television or newspapers can drop in from afar onto the patch, to write and broadcast without the responsibility of living in the local community, or needing to return for your help with stories. The local journalists are here alongside you all the time, which means that while we will always try and tell it as it is, we're keen to give all sides a fair hearing, because we **will** want your help in the future.

Certainly at Ashworth nowadays, there has been a real attempt to discard that automatic reaction, as it sometimes appeared to us, to restrict to the minimum the information given to us. Things do go wrong, but when an organisation holds its hands up to it, then an informed journalist, who knows the place already, and has a professional relationship with the hospital, will be much more understanding and less likely to give the story the shock-horror spin. But you need to do this on the basis of a clearly defined agenda, led by the director of communications and agreed at board level. It should not merely be on the hoof.

To go back to the case of the rooftop protest when our reporter was asked to leave. A rooftop protest isn't, as I said earlier, necessarily a negative story, as Ashworth's initial silence seemed to imply. As I now know, the reality of rooftop protests at Ashworth is that the design of the wards makes access to the roof all too easy. So, while on the one hand, journalists believed this to be a rarity; on the other hand, the hospital did not see it as much out of the ordinary.

Nevertheless, how much better for Ashworth to have realised it could be seen as a story and leaked by some member of staff with a grudge to bear. They could have alerted us to the facts (in the context of it not being a unique occurrence) and so been able to emphasise the speed of their response and effective management of the situation, rather than their lack of control in allowing the protest to have happened at all.

If there were concerns about those on the roof having radios, we are going to respect those concerns, and we will certainly restrict what we broadcast — but we need to be trusted — for better or worse. If we misuse that trust, then we know that we will not be in a good position to get help from you in the future.

Now, it's true that our reporter wanted to be allowed inside the hospital, but, equally, we knew that was unlikely to be granted. Perhaps, though, he could have been given a cup of tea, given some background information, even though the hospital was aware he was on a fruitless quest, rather than being ordered off the premises. At the very least, they might have got one journalist slightly more on-side than he would otherwise have been.

As regards the hostage incident, the same thing applies. If there are genuine reasons why we cannot see the report, tell us what those reasons are; if possible, give us edited versions; but whatever you do, get your case across **before** anyone else manages to put you on the defensive.

Although it has got a great deal better, the lessons have not as yet been fully learnt. On one occasion, *The Mirror* newspaper got hold of an exclusive about Ashworth — and that means that someone leaked it for one of the reasons that I've given. The truth of the story was that a couple of weapons were very nearly — if unintentionally — taken in a suitcase onto a ward at the hospital by a patient. Management should have realised the story was going to be leaked and they should have managed it. The fact was that the security systems worked, at least the failsafe did, because the weapons **were** discovered, even though it was at the security area at ward level. And it could have been made clear that the patient in question, was **not** trying 'to get weapons into Ashworth', as the Liverpool *Daily Post* headlined it. The media would have been told that the weapons were in fact two unusable air guns and that the patient had not got a clue what was in the suitcase, one of six cases he was collecting from his sister's house, where they had been stored for ten years, because she was moving into an old people's home.

Certainly there had been a series of failures, including no search at the sister's home, nor at the two security gates, but if it had been the hospital which had informed the press — the broadsheets, rather than the tabloids —I would suggest then the *Mirror* would have lost its exclusive tag; it would be less likely to have described the patient as a 'dangerman'; that a notorious child murderer was on the same ward, which was totally irrelevant to the story, and might have been played down. In addition, the *Mirror* would probably not have solicited ludicrous quotes from an unnamed source. These included, 'if the patients had got hold of any of the weapons, they could have tried to escape or held prison officers hostage'.

If management doesn't grasp the nettle and get to the press before the troublemakers put an unhelpful spin on events, then time and energy will continue to be wasted defending disinformation. Somehow or other, you need to spot the problems, whatever they are, and control the release of information before someone else gets to the media first. If you can manage that, I think you'll be pleasantly surprised at the results. Of course there are problems of patient confidentiality, but I suspect that 'patient confidentiality' is routinely used to protect management failure more than anything else. I believe there can be ways round it, if need be.

To my mind, the fundamental issue is defusing the aura of secrecy still hanging over all special hospitals. And to be fair, it's a secrecy that is very understandable: the hospital is often in a 'Catch-22' situation. On the one hand, society (and, indeed, some professionals) say lock these people up and throw away the key; on the other hand, there is a prurient interest in them, and a sort of perverse glee, usually dressed up as moral outrage, when things, as they always will, go wrong. Certainly, that dilemma meant that Ashworth used to sometimes get caught in a mind-set that led to silly decisions.

For instance, one of the national papers reported that a patient, who had attracted considerable publicity, was no longer at Ashworth. We checked and were told that no comment was possible. Staff are frequently asked about this patient, whose name is often mentioned in the media, including calls about the hospital on my programme.

Why the 'no comment'? The reality was that if the patient had been moved, the story would have eventually come out; so why not have taken control and released it officially or knocked the story on the head? As usual, patient confidentiality was the excuse. If there is a good reason that the public is not to know something, tell us that reason. The public has a right to be given information, however much some might personally dislike the attitude they have in response to that information. Any part of a mental health service needs to be aware of the public's perceptions and not hide from them, but, whenever possible, explain what's happening; and, if the public view is based on misinformation, correct that misinformation.

At the root of the public misconceptions of Ashworth is the lack of understanding that it's a hospital — part of the National Health Service, the NHS, and not a prison — that it's dealing with very sick people. That is the challenge that Ashworth faces, and that it has been trying to confront for the last decade.

The documentary mentioned earlier, *Taking Out the Stitches*, about the high dependency women's ward, is a good example of Ashworth facing up to the challenge of being pro-active — and maybe helped some of the staff have pride in their work. There was enormous nervousness about us making the programme, the aim of which was to capture a day in the life of the ward. We would normally spend a couple of days recording anything and everything that went on, and talking to those people who wished to be interviewed. I think we would have produced a far better programme had we done just that. But there was not enough trust to allow us to be free to record what we wished, and then to have got subsequent agreements from individuals and consultants as to which material we could and could not use. On the other hand, we were allowed to interview one patient who hadn't previously agreed to talk, but who changed her mind while we were there, and retrospective permission from her consultant was obtained.

We also wanted to be able to talk to any patients who agreed, about their past history and why they were in Ashworth. However, that was ruled out of bounds, even though I believe we could have got round the obvious problems of confidentiality of patients and their relatives, and concern for their victims. From the little we did learn during our recording there, we know that some of the women's past experiences would have allowed the public a much deeper understanding of, and perhaps even sympathy with, the patients, and with the difficulties faced by the staff at Ashworth.

I do not believe that the public is as unsympathetic as some in the mental health service fear — but, in any case, the public cannot understand what the public doesn't know. Of course, I am not suggesting that you should exploit the patients just to get the hospital's message across, but I say to Ashworth and to everyone working with the mentally ill, especially mentally ill offenders — be even bolder than you are, and think about how you can ultimately help all your patients by working with the media with the agreement of some of them. Much of this applies to staff and managers working in other areas of health care.

One Ashworth chief executive was truly bold: she invited Channel 4 to make a fly-on-the-wall documentary about the changes that she intended to make. She knew the difficulties that lay ahead and she knew that there was no point in hiding those difficulties. Indeed, there was every reason to let the public know and understand what was happening, and to publicise the quality of much of the work that goes on there.

Unfortunately, it was, in my view, partly the fear of that documentary from some of the staff, which led to her authority being undermined and to her consequent resignation. But she was right. And she was also right to have realised that internal and external communications did not simply mean having a press officer. One important legacy of her tenure was the appointment of a director of communications at board level, with a wide-ranging brief to turn around Ashworth's image with the staff, the public, civil servants and ministers — indeed, within the health service as a whole — putting education, in its broadest sense, at the heart of Ashworth, and not shying away from the truth, good, bad and ugly, for better or for worse. That new post is a major part of the reasons for the improvements I've outlined. In my view, one should, together with the staff, circumspectly stop hiding one's lights and dark corners under a bushel. In truth, you have much to be proud of, and anything you have to hide will, in any event, get out. Oscar Wilde suggested, 'If one tells the truth, one is sure sooner or later to be found out' (Wilde, 1987).

Develop relationships with individual journalists, particularly local journalists, as the chief executive and her team did with me. There will always be those inside and outside any institution who don't wish you well, and there will always be lousy journalists, but don't leave the field to them. Take the initiative, defuse the mystery of the institution, open up in every way. Be honest about the good, the bad and the ugly, until Ashworth, or whatever aspect of health care you are involved with, becomes properly understood as a place of care, where containment is needed to give that proper care. A place with nurses, not prison officers; with patients, not inmates; a hospital, not a prison. Only then will there be a real chance of creating caring communities, within and without the walls.

Key points

❋ Groups which are traditionally reviled by the public can receive a fairer representation in the press, if managers and those in charge develop an individual relationship with journalists.

❋ There are many examples, past and present, of stigmatisation of mental health service users in the media. However, journalists have also stimulated Government inquiries to effect improvements and worked proactively with health service participants. The latter can result in accounts which empower service users and carers.

❋ The media and particularly local radio can be used effectively, both to reach people served by a health service and to engender pride.

❋ Giving no information is more likely to result in journalists assuming a 'cover up', with the reporting of stories which reflect individuals' interests and prejudices. It also results in time wasted 'defending disinformation', with lost opportunities to enable better public understanding of patients' perspectives.

❋ Ashworth's positive, pro-active attempts to work with the media included the appointment of a press and public relations officer, an invitation to the author to visit the hospital and a public exhibition of patients' art. This contrasts with examples of unproductive decisions to give no information at all.

❋ 'Horror stories' about Ashworth have sometimes been published. Staff members' leaks to the press may be prevented through in-house education; and giving the media, and thus, the public, appropriate information. If a health service works proactively with a journalist, and is honest in giving information about any mistakes, (s)he is less likely to produce 'horror stories'.

❋ In certain circumstances, confidentiality should not be used as a reason for not giving journalists information. Reasons for not giving the public certain information need to be explained.

References

Angermeyer MC, Matschinger H (1996) The effect of violent attacks by schizophrenic persons on the attitude of the public towards the mentally ill. *Soc Sci and Med* **43**(12): 1721–8

Blom-Cooper, Sir L, Brown M, Dolan K, Murphy E (1992) Great Britain HM Government. Department of Health Report of the Committee of Inquiry into Complaints about Ashworth Hospital. CM 20280. HMSO, London

Collins M (1999) The practitioner new to the role of forensic psychiatric nurse in the UK. In: Robinson D, Kettles A, eds. *Forensic Nursing and Multidisciplinary Care of the Mentally Disordered Offender*. Jessica Kingsley, London

Department of Health (1999) *Managing dangerous people with a severe personality disorder proposals for policy development*. HMSO, London

Oliver M, Barnes C (1998) *Disabled People and Social Policy*. Longman, London

Pilgrim D, Waldron L (1998) User involvement in mental health service developments. How far can it go? *J Mental Health* **1**: 95–104

Sayce L (2000) *From Psychiatric Patient to Citizen. Overcoming Discrimination and Social Exclusion*. Macmillan, Basingstoke

Shalala DE (1999) Secretary of Health and Human Services, *Unpublished Conference Speech*. The White House

Stone H (1969) Introductory notes on Dickens C and Wills WH 'A Curious Dance Round a Curious Tree'. In: Stone H, ed. (1969) *The Uncollected Writings of Charles Dickens. Household Words, 1850–1859 Volume 2*. Allen Lane/Penguin, London: 381–91

Wilde O (1987) *The Works of Oscar Wilde. Phrases and philosophies for the use of the young, 1894*. Galley Press/WH Smith, Leicester: 1113

19

The creative arts and empowerment

Jackie Green and Keith Tones

Introduction

The arts have a unique capacity to engage with our feelings. There can be few of us who have not experienced the 'feel good factor' that contact with the arts can bring. In a very general way, the arts can contribute to a positive sense of well-being and, if health is defined holistically, to overall health status. The arts can also be used to enhance communication at a number of levels. At the most basic, this might simply involve increasing aesthetic appeal or lending clarity. At a more sophisticated level, the arts can rouse emotions and contribute to empathic understanding. The arts have been widely used to make political statements. Theatre is notable in this sphere, but there are numerous other examples ranging from Shostakovitch symphonies to the protest songs of the 1970s, from Picasso's Guernica to the work of Damien Hirst. The words of the Russian poet Vladimir Mayakovsky, 'art is not a mirror to reflect the world, but a hammer with which to shape it' emphasise the potential role of the arts in raising awareness of oppression and social inequality and motivating people to take action. Such action might well be directed towards achieving health goals through addressing the social and environmental determinants of health.

In contrast to this general and perhaps incidental impact on health status, the arts have been put to more explicit use in the health context. Initially, their use principally centred on art as therapy. More recently the arts have been used in health promotion to achieve both disease prevention and more salutogenic goals. The focus of this chapter is on the use of arts to promote health and well-being at both an individual and community level, and particularly their contribution to individual and community empowerment. The features of such 'arts for health' projects, which distinguish them from the more general contribution of the arts to health, include participation and active involvement in the creative process — hence the frequent use of the term 'creative arts' in this context.

During the last decade there has been a rapid expansion in the number of community-based 'arts for health' projects. Some evidence of the mainstreaming of this type of work is provided by recent developments such as the establishment of the Institute of Medical Humanities; the setting up of the Centre for Arts and Humanities in Health and Medicine (http://www.dur.ac.uk/cahhm); and the Health Development Agency maintaining a website on arts and community participation for health (http://www.artsncommunities.hda-online.org.uk). Anticipated benefits from the work of the Institute include:

- more compassionate, intuitive doctors and other health practitioners
- improved patient empowerment through creative expression
- reduced dependence on antidepressant and anxiolytic medication, and enhanced confidence, self-reliance and mental health of individuals and communities and reduced social exclusion (Baum and Philipp, 2000).

The policy context

The WHO position on health promotion has consistently emphasised the importance of:

- equity
- empowerment
- active community participation (WHO, 1986; WHO, 1997).

Recent developments in health policy in the UK (DoH, 1999) have also focused on tackling inequality and social exclusion and emphasised the importance of involving local communities in partnerships to improve health and build social capital.

The Alma Ata conference (WHO, 1978) recognised the central role of primary health care. Despite calls for a re-orientation of health care to address the determinants of health (WHO, 1986), primary care in the developed world has remained essentially concerned with an individualised approach to disease management and prevention. The structural changes introduced by the *New NHS* (DoH, 1997) have placed primary care in a key position through the creation of primary care groups and trusts. The role of primary care has been extended beyond providing personal health care to include improving the health of the community. The development of this broader public health function demands a shift from a narrow biomedical focus on the individual towards involving communities in identifying their health needs and working with other sectors to build 'healthy alliances' to promote health. In short, it involves a shift from reactive to pro-active work and a refocusing of effort 'upstream'. This new approach offers opportunities, but also presents many challenges. Peckham (1998), for example, notes that:

> *GPs, despite some heroic exceptions, are not known for their skills in collaboration or for their appreciation of the potential contribution of their patients.*

Clearly these developments call for new styles of working. Similarly, other initiatives and structures which have recently emerged, such as healthy living centres, health action zones and health improvement plans, also demand innovative approaches. The use of creative arts or 'arts for health' projects offers considerable potential for responding to these new challenges as well as contributing to individual health.

Arts for health projects

The variety and scope of 'arts for health' projects is limited only by the imagination of people involved — and the availability of funding and resources. Some examples of the ways in which the arts have been used to promote health are provided below and derive from a case study of the use of creative arts in an innovative general practice (Tones and Green, 1999; Rigler, 1996). While it is impossible, in this short space, to do full justice to the creativity of individuals working with the creative arts, the selection will provide a flavour of the diversity of projects.

Writer in residence in the surgery

A professional writer worked with patients to encourage them to write accounts of their own experience of illness. Such accounts were compiled into a book and made available for other patients to read.

Artist in residence in the surgery

A teacher was seconded from a local school to work with patients and the various artefacts produced were displayed in the surgery.

Immunisation parties

A number of factors led to the development of this initiative, including: concern that the experience of having an injection might make children fearful of coming to the surgery; the availability of an anaesthetising cream and the need to occupy the children during the time it took to work; and, low uptake of immunisation. The immunisation sessions were structured to have a party atmosphere and included story-telling and colouring sheets all based on the theme of Harold the Hedgehog, who had lost one of his spikes and needed to have it put back. A larger than life Harold was in attendance and a flexible castle was constructed in part of the surgery as his home. Pupils and the art teacher from a local secondary school were involved in designing and constructing these materials, providing childcare and background music — activities which fitted in with their school course-work.

Needs assessment

Staff from a further education college set up an art project in a primary school involving the children, their parents and grandparents and also pupils from the local secondary school. People were encouraged to express their views about health and the community through the medium of art. The secondary pupils were also asked to put their ideas into words. The overall picture which emerged graphically revealed fear of crime and going out at night; the problem of traffic; and the issue of loneliness.

Artists in residence in a school

Artists worked with pupils on the theme of lungs, fresh air, and the joy of breathing and the problems of environmental pollution and smoking. A series of posters were produced which were used in the local surgery and also made available nationally together with a series of post cards. A giant mobile was constructed and installed in the school entrance hall and a 'lung box' was developed for use as a visual aid in the surgery to demonstrate the effects of smoking.

Street theatre

School staff and a theatre company worked with secondary school pupils to develop a production which would improve public understanding of the immune system and reduce unnecessary demand for antibiotics. Performances, which took the form of an interactive game show, were given in the local shopping centre and primary schools and were well received.

Lantern procession

The lantern procession was developed as a response to the social isolation in a community. Lantern making workshops were led by a professional artist in the surgery and local schools in the period before the 'festival'. The event itself was highly symbolic — there was a procession around the local houses, lighting the streets and drawing people out of the isolation of their houses, culminating in a party. From small beginnings in 1990 with only fifteen families taking part, it became an annual tradition and by 1996, there were 400 families involved.

The range of examples demonstrates some variation both in the degree of participation and creativity required. The relevance of some of these projects to health is immediately evident whereas for others — and, indeed, for the sceptical — it is rather more tenuous. Furthermore, at first sight, some of the projects appear to be focused on biomedical goals, whereas others are more holistic in approach. For example, the use of Harold the Hedgehog parties to increase the uptake of immunisation would be entirely consistent with conventional preventive health goals. This type of approach can also contribute to the empowerment and salutogenic goals described in Tones and Green (2002). A particular feature of the creative arts is their capacity to operate at multiple levels and achieve multiple goals. The influence of 'arts for health' projects on the various constructs of individual and community empowerment will now be explored, together with the complex interactions.

Individual empowerment and the creative arts

One of the more obvious ways in which creative arts projects can contribute to health is by enhancing health-related learning, which has been defined by Tones and Tilford (1994, p. 11) as, 'a relatively permanent change in an individual's capability or disposition'.

Learning outcomes might therefore include:

• knowledge and understanding
• beliefs and values
• attitudes and emotional states
• skills.

For example, projects which involve people in developing educational materials — of whatever form, from posters and leaflets, through to artworks and drama performances — will **enhance the learning** of those taking part. This is aptly summarised in the aphorism *docendo discimus* — we learn by teaching. The process may also involve the development of skills which, together with the tangible evidence provided by the successful production of materials, will contribute to **self-efficacy beliefs, confidence and a sense of control**. Clearly, if the 'products' are valued by others, then there will be further enhancement of self-esteem. All these various impacts have been identified in Tones and Green (2002), as constructs of individual empowerment. If those involved feel that they are achieving worthwhile goals, then the **meaningfulness** of their involvement will lead to an enhanced **sense of coherence** (Antonovsky, 1984). The outcomes will contribute to both individual empowerment and a sense of coherence, which might be viewed as worthwhile goals in their own right. However, people with a strong sense of coherence are more likely to remain healthy and, empowered individuals are more likely to take action to prevent ill health.

A key question concerns the subsequent use of any educational materials developed. Strictly, this in itself would not come under the umbrella of creative arts, although the meaningfulness of the creative arts project which produced them would be heavily dependent on the use to which they were put and the way in which they were received. The effectiveness and relevance of the materials is likely to be enhanced by the fact that they were produced locally by people with whom the recipient identifies.

This conforms with the principle of **homophily** (Rogers and Shoemaker, 1971) which suggests that people are more likely to believe and respond to messages from people with whom they identify closely.

The experience of ill-health can itself be depowering through feelings of loss of control. Projects encouraging creative writing about the experience of illness, referred to above, can help to restore a sense of control, and even mastery, by enabling patients to explore and articulate their feelings. Publishing these locally authored accounts for other patients to read can also help them to overcome feelings of isolation and, at a more practical level, establish support networks. Even relatively simple initiatives such as involving patients in the design and refurbishment of waiting rooms can convey the message that patients are valued partners. Similarly, the layout of waiting areas and display of materials and artefacts can encourage communication and reflect concern with well-being.

> *The creation of decorations not only makes the waiting room more pleasant to be in, it subtly alters the way patients and staff see the surgery itself. It ceases to be the territory of experts and becomes a public space which can reflect the community's own perceptions of themselves and their world.*

> (McDonnell, undated, p. 10)

Participation in creative arts projects can bring people into contact with social networks and also help to develop and consolidate the latter networks. Membership of such networks enhances the sense of self and self-esteem. Furthermore, access to support helps individuals to feel that their lives are manageable and contributes to a sense of coherence. There is clearly some overlap and reciprocity between individual and community empowerment which will be discussed more fully below.

Perhaps the most graphic way of encapsulating the benefits to individuals deriving from their participation in 'arts for health' projects is through their own words:

> *I now tackle things I would never have thought of doing before... it has made me stronger.*

> (Mrs White)

> *... the sense of satisfaction that the arts work gave me, made me value me for the first time. This made me able to do things — only on a small front — like make decisions that I would've taken ages to make. Because I could see something I had created, it makes me think I can do things in my life, that before I had not control over. I haven't changed the world, but I'm doing little things for me, like*

*writing to shops to complain, to the bus station about the
lack of buses, things like that.*

(Mrs Red, Durrant, 1993, p. 105)

Community empowerment and the creative arts

An active empowered community is not merely a group of empowered
individuals. There also needs to be a 'sense of community'. McMillan
and Chavis (1986, p. 9) identify the main elements of a sense of
community as:

* ❖ Membership — a feeling of belonging.
* ❖ Influence — '... of making a difference to the group and of the
  group mattering to its members'.
* ❖ Integration and fulfilment of needs — '... a feeling that members'
  needs will be met by the resources received through their
  membership in the group'.
* ❖ Shared emotional connection — '... the commitment and belief
  that members have shared and will share history, common places,
  time together, and similar experiences'.

Reference to the description of a sense of coherence in Tones and
Green (2002) will demonstrate some commonalities with the
constructs of a sense of community. A number of different types of
creative arts projects have been used to develop a sense of community.
The lantern festival referred to above provides a useful illustration.
The location for this initiative was a rapidly developing housing
estate, which lacked the infrastructure to support social cohesion.
There was an influx of newcomers, many of whom worked outside
the area. Given this context, it is hardly surprising that there was little
sense of community and that loneliness and isolation were rife.
Preparation for the festival brought people together in a mutually
dependent way — everyone's contribution mattered. People developed
skills in making lanterns and all the other tasks required to make the
event happen successfully, which boosted their own confidence and
self-efficacy beliefs. They also passed on these skills to others. The
contacts and networks built up then provided an on-going source of
more general information and support. In addition to the symbolic
role of the procession itself in drawing people out of the isolation of

their homes, it became an annual event — a shared tradition.

Where there are well established social networks, they are frequently used for informal support and advice — the so-called lay referral system. In the absence of such networks, it is often left to professional agencies, such as the health service, to take on this role. This has two main repercussions. On the one hand, it can lead to inappropriate use of services. On the other, it contributes to the progressive medicalisation of life first referred to by Illich (1976) and the gradual erosion of a community's capacity to deal with its problems.

There is a considerable body of evidence to suggest that social connectedness and social support has a positive effect on health and well-being. The mechanism of action is not clearly understood — access to lay referral systems and practical support may be part of, but not the whole answer, and emotional resources are also felt to be important. Wilkinson and Marmot (1998, p. 21) summarise the role of social support:

> *Support operates on the levels of both the individual and the society. Social isolation and exclusion are associated with increased rates of premature death and poorer chances of survival after a heart attack. People who get less emotional and social support from others are more likely to experience less well-being, more depression, a greater risk of pregnancy complications and higher levels of disability from chronic diseases. In addition, the bad aspects of close relationships can lead to poor mental and physical health. ... Social cohesion — the existence of mutual trust and respect in the community and wider society — helps to protect people and their health. ... One study of a community with high levels of social cohesion showed low rates of coronary heart disease, which increased when social cohesion in the community declined.*

The concept of 'social capital' as developed by Putnam (1993a; 1993b) refers to the level of cohesion within a community and its capacity to act co-operatively to tackle local problems. Cooper *et al* (1999, p. 7) suggest that it includes all the 'social, collective, economic and cultural resources to which the community or population has access'. The potential of the creative arts to develop social capital can readily be identified within Gillies' (1997) characterisation of communities with high levels of social capital as having:

- high levels of trust
- positive social norms
- many overlapping and diverse horizontal networks for communication and exchange of information, ideas and practical help.

Social and environmental factors exert an important influence on health. Even if there is a strong sense of community and high levels of social capital, a community will only be prompted to challenge the factors which adversely affect its members' health if there is also:

- awareness of the issue
- motivation to take action.

The term 'critical consciousness raising', which is associated with the work of the educationalist Paulo Freire, can be applied to the process of addressing both these points. Freire's (1972) approach involves four stages:

- reflection on personal reality
- exploration and collective identification of the root causes of that reality
- examination of implications
- planning action to change reality.

Such planning and action based on critical reflection was referred to as praxis by Freire. People must also believe that it is possible to achieve change and that they have the skills to do it. Although the roots of this approach are in participative (and liberatory) education, the creative arts can also contribute to critical reflection on reality. Theatre, in particular, has been much used for this purpose. The fellow Brazilian, Augusto Boal, developed a form of theatre often known as 'forum theatre'. Members of the audience with ideas for change could go on stage to act out their ideas — the audience was transformed from spectators to 'spect-actors'. Boal observed that such participation enabled the audience to imagine change, act it out and then reflect collectively on the change. The further observation that this empowered the audience to take social action led to the use of this type of theatre as a vehicle for social change, the so-called 'Theatre of the Oppressed' (Paterson, 1999).

Both the process and the outcomes of working for social change can be empowering. Clearly, if the social and environmental conditions are oppressive, then action to tackle the causes of that oppression will lead to an environment which in itself is more empowering. Moreover, the experience of success, however small, will boost the confidence, self-esteem and sense of control of those involved and make it more likely that they will take up other causes. The vicious circle of learned helplessness can gradually be turned round into a virtuous circle of participation and empowerment. The importance of past success is recognised by Putnam (1995, p. 67, cited in Cooper *et al*, 1999):

> *At the same time, networks of civic engagement embody past success at collaboration, which can serve as a cultural template for future collaboration. Finally, the dense networks of interaction probably broaden the participants' sense of self, developing the 'I' into the 'we'... '.*

The relationship between individual empowerment, a sense of community and community empowerment is complex and all these elements add to the stock of social capital. The creative arts have enormous potential to influence the various components in a mutually reinforcing way as summarised in *Figure 19.1*.

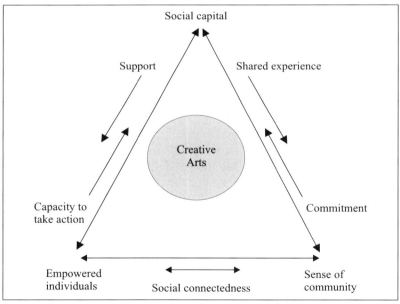

Figure 19.1: The contribution of creative arts to individual and community empowerment

Needs assessment

In contrast to the grassroots social activism just described, the importance of 'listening to local voices' and tapping into the reserves of lay knowledge and experience (Williams and Popay, 1994) is receiving increased recognition by those in power. Community development is one way of ensuring that people are heard:

A process by which ordinary people can have some say in prioritising, planning, delivering and reviewing services.

(UK Health for All Network, 1993)

The restructuring of the NHS and the creation of the internal market focused attention on the identification of need as a basis for commissioning services. Bradshaw's well-known taxonomy identifies four different needs:

- normative — based on professional judgement
- comparative — based on comparison with other groups or areas
- felt — identified by members of the community
- expressed — articulation of felt needs by words actions or other means.

(Bradshaw, 1972)

The felt needs of the community are clearly of central importance. The expression of these needs in a systematic way will, however, be dependent on the creation of appropriate opportunities to facilitate the process. The creative arts have a valuable role. They put people in touch with their feelings and enable them to express them in often graphic and moving ways. By engaging the imagination, the arts allow people to see how things might be rather than becoming inured to how they are. The needs assessment project described earlier, which culminated in a display of the artwork of different generations depicting their community, revealed a picture aptly summarised by the arts adviser as 'chilling'. It communicated the message to local policy makers more clearly and possibly, more powerfully, than through any other medium.

Further examples of the use of creative arts as a vehicle for exploring need are provided by McDonnell (undated). In response to epidemiological evidence that there was an increase in teenage pregnancy (normative and comparative need) a theatre group was commissioned to work with young people to explore their needs (enabling them to express their felt needs). A theatre production was developed and following the performance the audience was engaged in debate. The issues that emerged included:

- young people finding the literature used for sex education boring and alienating
- using the surgery clinic for contraceptive advice made them feel exposed as they could be seen by people they knew
- lack of liaison between schools and medical services.

Understanding the situation from the standpoint of young people resulted in improvements in service provision.

Evaluation and good practice

Those who have been directly involved in 'arts for health' projects have witnessed the empowering transformations that can take place at both individual and community level. Along with the general move to evidence-based practice, there is some pressure to demonstrate effectiveness and to learn lessons from experience. The previous sections have attempted to demonstrate from a theoretical perspective how the creative arts can influence the constructs of individual and community empowerment. The Health Education Authority's (HEA; now Health Development Agency [HDA]) review of good practice in community-based 'arts for health' projects noted that evaluations which address health criteria were rare (HEA, 1999). Furthermore, project workers were often concerned about the possibly reductionist nature of evaluation. However, the summary bulletin proposes a broad range of outcome indicators including:

- enhanced motivation (within the project and in participants' lives generally)
- greater social connectedness
- people's perceptions that they have a more positive outlook on life
- reduced sense of fear, isolation and anxiety
- increased confidence, sociability and self-esteem.

The review identified participation as a pivotal link between the arts activities and health outcomes and saw the principal gains as:

- development of inter-personal skills
- opportunities to make new friends
- increased involvement.

(HEA, 1999)

A study undertaken by Comedia (Matarasso, 2001), generated a list of some fifty social impacts deriving from participation in arts projects. A number of them are concerned with educational opportunity, development of skills and increased employability. While all fifty will impact on empowerment in some way, the following selection is perhaps of particular relevance:

- increase people's confidence and sense of self-worth
- provide a forum to explore personal rights and responsibilities
- reduce isolation by helping people make friends
- develop community networks and sociability
- build community organisational capacity
- encourage local self-reliance and project management
- help people extend control over their own lives
- be a means of gaining insight into political and social ideas
- facilitate effective public consultation and participation
- strengthen community co-operation and networking
- help feel a sense of belonging and involvement
- create community tradition in new towns or neighbourhoods
- help community groups to raise their vision beyond the immediate.

Although it focused primarily on educational outcomes, a recent study conducted by the National Foundation for Educational Research (NFER, 2000), identified a number of benefits of good and effective arts teaching in schools which are also of relevance to health and include:

- heightened enjoyment and fulfilment
- increase in knowledge
- personal and social development
- skill development:
  - communication and expression
  - thinking skills
  - creativity.

Tones and Green (1999) noted the central importance of the commitment, vision and enthusiasm of key individuals in setting up 'arts for health' projects and the need to involve skilled individuals in operationalising the project. The HEA's review of good practice (1999) also endorsed this. The review noted that, 'there is no one single winning formula' (p. 4) for 'arts for health' projects and made a number of recommendations. Access to good quality space is important both for producing and displaying or performing the art-work, but also to facilitate informal contact on a 'drop-in' basis. The value of participation has already been noted. However, the quality of the artwork itself was found to be equally important and to influence the extent to which the participants take the work seriously; have a pride in it; and, feel they can use the medium to express themselves. Adopting a rigorous approach to teaching basic skills (and when necessary, correcting them) was not seen to be in conflict with participatory approaches, but rather as instrumental to achieving high quality outcomes. The participatory models that worked best were 'well-structured, well-organised and specifically related to the acquisition of skills or of resources for self-expression' (HEA, 1999, p. 5). Clearly, funding is an issue and the report recommends wider dissemination of possible sources of funding together with three-year funding packages to allow adequate time for project development. The report concludes that, 'there is growing recognition of the need to make arts projects a mainstream part of larger initiatives, such as health action zones or healthy living centres' (p. 4). The evidence from robust evaluations can only add to that recognition.

The Declaration of Windsor (1998) *Arts, Health and Well-Being: Beyond the Millenium — The Role of Humanities in Medicine* endorsed the importance of ethics and the humanities in: medical education; public health; community development; caring for people; and, promoting better health and well-being. A twelve-point action plan was produced, including:

❖ 'Produce a 'user's guide' to the practice and benefits of arts in health care and healthy living initiatives for NHS managers responsible for budgeting and commissioning services.

❖ Publish other documents on the vital contribution of arts and design in hospitals, surgeries and other healthcare settings, outlining the cost-effectiveness and the potential of improving the quality of life for patients, visitors, staff and the surrounding community.

❖ Catalogue the qualitative and quantitative research evidence, create a taxonomy of the field; list relevant professional associations and organisations specialising in arts in health.

❖ Promote the notion of arts as a means of self-expression and a catalyst for strengthening and energising communities and enhancing the psychological, physical and emotional health and well-being of the individuals who make up those communities.

❖ Revive and promote the notion of 'healthy living centres' such as the Pioneer Health Centre in Peckham, London, so that arts activity may become woven into the fabric of everyday life; and 'to maintain and extend skills of those who practise arts therapy and promote the recreational value of arts to health' (Nuffield Trust, 1999).

Many of today's health problems are the product of social inequality and social exclusion. Responding to these problems and making a more positive contribution to individual and community empowerment requires 'a prescription of ideas not medicine' (Rigler, in Tones and Green, 1999, p. 18). The creative arts offer us a plethora of such ideas.

Key points

⌘ The arts can help people to get in touch with feelings, enable communication; and 'make political statements... raising awareness of oppression and social inequality and motivating people to take action.'

⌘ Within health services, the arts have been used both therapeutically, and in health promotion, with an increasing number of 'arts for health' projects and supporting organisations.

⌘ Both the World Health Organization and the Department of Health have been concerned to reduce 'inequality and social exclusion'. Recent Department of Health policy is concerned with enabling communities to identify and promote 'their health needs'.

⌘ Arts for health projects help to achieve this. Examples include a writer and an artist in general practices, 'immunisation parties' for children, arts projects in schools, street theatre and a lantern festival.

⌘ Reported benefits of the arts in health care, include health education, skills development contributing to 'self-efficacy beliefs, confidence and a sense of control'; and for some individuals, increases in self-esteem, meaningfulness and a 'sense of coherence'. Opportunities for expression and decreased isolation have also been reported. In one project, artists worked with school pupils to produce health education materials.

⌘ Creative arts can also increase community empowerment. For example, a lantern festival enabled the sharing of skills, established links between people, and led to further support, and the establishment of 'a shared tradition'. Research findings suggest that health is enhanced by cohesive social networks, and accessible social and other resources ('social capital') When these are absent, there can be an over-reliance on professional advice and support.

⌘ The use of the arts in healthcare can also result in 'critical consciousness raising', enabling participants to reflect on, and change aspects of unhealthy environments, enabling the latter to be 'more empowering'. Success in achieving change increases individual empowerment and participation.

⌘ People in power are increasingly 'listening to local voices'. The arts can be used in community development: to convey messages in vivid ways to policy makers, and influence service provision. An example is the use of theatre to explore young people's expressed needs related to sex education literature and contraception; and thus, improve services in this area.

⌘ The Health Education Authority (1999) found that arts for health projects' own evaluations rarely addressed health criteria. 'The quality of ... artwork' was discovered to be as important as the opportunity to participate. Two other studies identified several positive outcomes relevant to empowerment and health. An action plan, produced in 1998, includes several suggestions for developing arts for health projects.

References

Antonovsky A (1984) The sense of coherence as a determinant of health. In: Matarazzo JD *et al*, eds. *Behavioral Health*. John Wiley, New York

Arts and Community Participation for Health online at: http://www.artsncommunities.hda-online.org.uk

Baum M, Philipp R (2000) New Institute of Medical Humanities in UK. *J Med Ethics: Medical Humanities* **26**: 63–4

Bradshaw J (1972) The concept of social need. *New Society* **19**(496): 640–3

Cooper H, Arber S, Fee L, Ginn J (1999) *The Influence of Social Support and Social Capital on Health: a review and analysis of British data.* HEA, London

Department of Health (1999) *Saving Lives: Our Healthier Nation.* DoH, London

Department of Health (1997) *The new NHS — modern, dependable.* DoH, London

Durrant K (1993) The Creative Arts and the Promotion of Health in Community Settings. MSc. dissertation, Leeds Metropolitan University

Freire P (1972) *Pedagogy of the Oppressed.* Penguin Books, Harmondsworth

Gillies P (1997) Social capital. *Healthlines* **45**: 15–17

Health Education Authority (1999) *Art for Health: a review of good practice in community-based arts projects and interventions which impact on health and well-being. Summary Bulletin.* HDA, London. Online at: http://www.hda-online.org.uk/pdfs/artforhealthsum.pdf

Illich I (1976) *The Limits of Medicine — Medical Nemesis: the Expropriation of Health.* Marion Boyars, London

McDonnell B (undated) *Serious Fun.* Dewsbury,Yorkshire and Humberside Arts

McMillan DW, Chavis DM (1986) Sense of community: a definition and theory. *J Community Psychol* **14**: 6–23

Matarasso F (2001) The health and social impact of participation in the arts. In: Heller T, Muston R, Sidell M, Lloyd C *Working for Health.* Sage, London

Medical Humanities online at: http://www.dur.ac.uk/cahhm

National Foundation for Educational Research (2000) *Arts Education in Secondary Schools: Effects and Effectiveness.* NFER, Slough

Nuffield Trust (1999) Declaration of Windsor. Online at: http://www.nuffieldtrust.org.uk/confer/conferb.htm (accessed 24/03/01)

Paterson D (1999) *Dr Augusto Boal: a Brief Biography.* Online at: http://www.unomaha.edu/~pto/augusto.htm (accessed 21/3/01)

Peckham S (1998) The missing link. *Health Service J*, 28 May: 22–3

Putnam RD, Leonardi R, Nanetti RY (1993a) *Making Democracy Work: Civic Traditions in Modern Italy.* Princeton University Press, Princeton, NJ

Putnam R (1993b) The prosperous community. *Am Prospect* **4**(13) Online at: http://www.prospect.org/print/\/4/13/putnam-r.html (accessed 23/03/01])

Rigler M (1996) *Withymoor Village Surgery — a Health Hive.* Dudley Priority Health NHS Trust, Dudley

Rogers EM, Shoemaker FF (1971) *Communication of Innovations.* Free Press, New York

Tones K, Green J (1999) *A Case Study of Withymoor Village Surgery — a Health Hive. Health Promotion and Creative Arts in General Practice.* Leeds Health Promotion Design, Leeds

Tones K, Green J (2002) The empowerment imperative in health promotion. In: Dooher J, Byrt R, eds. *Empowerment and Participation: Power, influence and control in contemporary health care.* Quay Books, Mark Allen Publishing Limited, Salisbury

Tones K, Tilford S (1994) *Health Education Effectiveness and Efficiency.* Chapman Hall, London

UK Health for All Network (1993) *Health for All Resource Pack.* UKHFAN, Liverpool

Wilkinson R, Marmot M, eds (1998) *The Solid Facts: the Social Determinants of Health.* WHO, Copenhagen

Williams G, Popay J (1994) Lay knowledge and the privilege of experience. In: Gabe J, Kelleher D, Williams G, eds. *Challenging Medicine.* Routledge, London

World Health Organization (1978) *Report on the International Conference on Primary Health Care. Alma Ata, 6–12 September.* WHO, Geneva

World Health Organization (1986) *Ottawa Charter for Health Promotion: an International Conference on Health Promotion.* WHO, Copenhagen

World Health Organization (1997) *The Jakarta Declaration on Leading Health Promotion into the 21st Century.* WHO, Geneva

20

Finding a voice: writing and empowerment

Mahendra Solanki and Richard Byrt

... I find my voice.
I speak... and my voice breathes new life to sustain me and
those I love.

(California Alliance for the Mentally Ill,
quoted in Fisher, 1999)

This chapter is concerned with the process of enabling patients in a medium secure unit, to 'find a voice': their own unique means of expression through creative writing.

In Autumn 1998, a group, consisting of a patient and staff of various disciplines, met to consider ways to increase further patients' creative activities involving the arts. A staff nurse suggested applying to the Poetry Places Scheme, funded by the Poetry Society. This scheme provides poets in residence to facilitate the writing and reading of poetry and make it accessible and relevant to individuals' lives. Participating organisations have included chain stores, schools, prisons and health service organisations (Sampson, 1999). As far as we know, Arnold Lodge is the first medium secure unit to receive a 'poetry place', but some mental health units and hospitals have been involved in this or similar programmes (McArdle and Byrt, 2001). This includes Rampton Hospital, where Benjamin Zephaniah has initiated poetry readings and workshops.

Establishing a writer in residence in a health service setting

In our experience, the following factors are essential in planning and initiating the work of a writer in residence, and in ensuring its success in empowering clients and patients in health service settings:

- establishing clients' needs
- enabling the writer in residence to be part of the organisation
- clarifying the aims of the residency

- establishing the extent and limits of client and professional power and participation in the organisation
- enlisting the support of organisational participants in positions of power
- the selection process
- communication with patients, managers and staff
- support, supervision and resources for the writer in residence.

The first part of this chapter will consider each of these factors in turn.

Establishing clients' needs

A writer in residence should be provided in response to clients' expressed wishes, rather than imposed by managers on reluctant clients. At Arnold Lodge, there was evidence of patients' needs for increased leisure activities in general, including activities involving the arts. In a patient satisfaction survey conducted with Leicestershire Community Health Council in 1998, social and recreational activities at evenings and weekends were lowly evaluated by patients, about half of whom rated these as 'quite bad' or 'very bad' (Leicestershire Community Health Council and Arnold Lodge, 1998). The appointment of a poet in residence (later a writer in residence) was one among several schemes to increase and improve leisure activities for patients. Other measures included the appointment of a social and recreational officer, establishing a committee, including patient representatives, to consider leisure activities; and the provision of the latter in response to patients' expressed preferences. Following these moves, there was a statistically significant increase in rated patient satisfaction in this area in the 2000 survey, compared with the previous year (Leicestershire Community Health Council and Arnold Lodge, 2000).

For several years, arts activities for patients, including creative writing and reading, had been introduced by Arnold Lodge staff and occasionally, outside facilitators. Informal feedback from several patients suggested that they had enjoyed these sessions. For this reason, and because of patients' expressed needs for additional leisure activities it was decided that an application to the poetry places scheme would be appropriate.

In the writer in residence's experience, one of the worst types of residency is where the poet is inflicted or imposed on unwilling subjects. This can be particularly the case in schools, where many children and young people report bad experiences of being forced to study literature, and poetry in particular. Their experience is reminiscent of poetry written by the Vogons in *The Hitch-hiker's Guide to the Galaxy*, this is described as the worst torture in the entire universe (Adams, 1979). If the impetus for creative writing comes from clients, rather than managers and staff, it is more likely to be perceived as positive, rather than a torment to be endured!

Enabling the writer in residence to be part of the organisation

For a residency to be successful, it is vital that the writer in residence is made welcome and is perceived to be a valued member of the health service organisation, and one who will contribute a fresh and different 'outsider' perspective. This involves his/her acceptance as a professional staff member who contributes to the clinical team, but is not involved in their day-to-day decisions.

In our experience, the extent to which health service clients and patients can use creative writing and reading in an empowering way depends, in part, on careful planning and communication. This is likely to be enhanced if one or more individuals are identified to co-ordinate and work with the writer in residence, in clarifying aims and arranging his/her induction and introduction to the organisation and its participants.

As soon as the Poetry Society notified Arnold Lodge that our bid to the Poetry Places scheme was successful, a staff member in the unit took on the role of 'co-ordinator' to liaise and communicate with managers and staff in the planning of the residency and its broad aims, the selection of the poet in residence and his introduction to the unit.

Enlisting the support of people with power

Within a collaborative, as opposed to an oppositional model, there is evidence that the success of attempts to increase participation and empowerment depends, in part, on the accurate, honest identification of individuals with power in the organisation; and the extent to which they are prepared to sanction proposals for client/patient participation and empowerment.

In order for the Arnold Lodge residency and its empowerment of patients to be successful, the co-ordinator considered it to be essential to work within a collaborative model; and to put forward initial proposals which would be likely to be acceptable to people with power in the organisation: ie. managers and senior staff such as consultant psychiatrists. Patients in secure units and hospitals have limited power because of their detention, often with Home Office restrictions, and the influence of current political, public and media demands for patients' incarceration (Lees and Withington, 2001).

From the outset, the idea of a writer in residence was well supported by managers. Planning the residency took particular account of the need to ensure the safety of patients and others and the security of the unit; and ways to facilitate the poet in residence's introduction to the unit and his work with patients. It was agreed that precise details of the work would be considered with the poet who was appointed and later, with patients. However, from the outset, and in response to the concerns of a few senior staff, it was decided to make clear that creative writing and reading would be provided as a leisure, rather than a therapeutic activity. It was made clear that the work would not constitute 'poetry therapy': the use of poetry as an adjunct to, or a form of psychotherapy (McArdle and Byrt, 2001). (This point is considered later in this chapter.)

In retrospect, more could have been done to consider the participation of patients and their views at this planning stage of the project. Some authors argue that participation is not meaningful or complete unless it involves clients/patients in the earliest stages (Ward, 2000, quoting Fleming and Ward, 1999). However, reports of participation of service users in research projects suggest that, in practice, 'differing levels of participation may occur at differing stages' (Kemshall and Littlechild, 2000, p. 236). In relation to the Arnold Lodge residency, participation was limited at the planning stage, partly because the co-ordinator did not want to raise patients' expectations in the event of a delay in the appointment or starting date of the writer in residence. In addition, within the constraints of time and other work, he considered it vital to concentrate his efforts on communicating with managers and staff, who had the power to agree to, or veto the project.

The selection process

In our experience, the selection process is another important factor in the success of a residency. The writer needs to have adequate information in order to establish whether (s)he is in broad agreement with the philosophy and aims of the organisation. Equally, organisational participants need to be sure that the writer in residence is likely to be sensitive to the needs of the clients and is able and willing to work within the organisation's philosophy and policies. On an initial visit, the writer needs the opportunity to meet as many organisational participants as possible. At Arnold Lodge, the writer in residence's first meeting was with several managers and staff of a variety of disciplines. We were fortunate that from the outset, there was commitment and enthusiasm on both sides to work together to enable patients to benefit from creative writing and reading.

Communication with patients, managers and staff

The careful communication of the appointment of a writer also appears to be vital to the success of a residency. Once the Arnold Lodge writer in residence was appointed, the co-ordinator communicated this to all patients, managers and staff. He arranged a carefully planned and thorough induction, in which the writer in residence was introduced to all patients and to staff and managers of **all** disciplines. Consequently, he soon became generally well known to everyone in the unit. The induction included consideration of the aims of the unit, issues concerning patients' assessment, care, treatment and rehabilitation, and the maintenance of safety. In the early days of the residency, the co-ordinator, who had some experience of facilitating creative writing with patients, accompanied the writer in residence to sessions, where this was considered necessary for safety reasons. Once his work was well established, the writer in residence received further induction and then saw patients individually, but with staff near at hand.

Good communication is essential to enable patients and staff to make plans and to feel comfortable with the writer in residence. It also aids the facilitation of relaxed sessions. In the early stages of the project, the co-ordinator informed patients, managers and staff of dates and times of sessions, both orally and in writing. This included the distribution of attractive posters of information for patients until the writer in residence was established in post and developed his own systems of communication.

We have found that communication with managers and funding bodies about the progress of projects and the numbers of patients attending is also important. Such reports can also provide material for applications for further funding; and as a basis for communicating details of the work through publication and conference presentations. This can contribute to the development of creative writing in other services.

Supervision, support and resources

In our experience, ongoing informal support and supervision need to be available to the writer in residence. Ideally, supervision needs to be both from someone within the organisation and (particularly for a writer who is new to the role) from an experienced writer in residence.

The writer in residence role requires flexibility and accommodation on the part of both writer and the organisation. The writer needs access to a desk, computer, telephone and stationery. Access to a quiet area for breaks and to food and beverages is especially important. A budget needs to be allocated to ensure that patients have access to a reasonably wide range of writing materials, books, magazines and recordings. Arnold Lodge patients have welcomed having a choice of A4 or A5 hard cover notebooks for their work, and for some individuals, access to computers.

Funding and the writer in residence's work

The identification of appropriate sources of funding is also important. The Poetry Society sponsored the first fifteen sessions of the writer in residence at Arnold Lodge. He has normally worked from about 2.00 pm to 9.00 pm, generally on a weekly basis, and has seen between twelve and fifteen individuals each week. Patients have a choice of individual or group sessions, with the majority choosing the former.

Informally, the sessions sponsored by the Poetry Society were positively evaluated by patients, managers and staff. For this reason, further funding was obtained firstly, from Central Nottinghamshire Healthcare Trust (which at the time, managed Arnold Lodge); and later, from a local charitable trust.

The writer in residence was originally known as a 'poet in residence' because of the initial funding from the Poetry Society's 'Poetry Places' scheme. However, once this funding ceased, he became known as a 'writer in residence' because this title better reflected his awareness of a need to broaden his role. This was in response to patients' wishes and the wide range and nature of their work. This has encompassed a rich diversity, including listening to, and writing song lyrics, serious and humorous poems, short stories, autobiographical accounts, the planning of a novel and conversation in Gujarati. The writer in residence has also provided input to educational assignments and the writing of letters. Patients who have worked with him range from individuals with undeveloped literacy skills to people who have been involved in creative writing for several years. Part of the work has involved a demystification of writing and reading, and enabling these activities to be accessible and enjoyable to individuals who have often had adverse school experiences.

The rest of this chapter will outline the process of facilitating creative writing and ways in which this empowers patients.

The need for flexibility and trust

It is important that the writer is sensitive to patients' particular perspectives and is prepared to be flexible in the way in which (s)he works and to accommodate change. It is vital that creative writing and reading are seen by patients to be accessible and relevant to their everyday lives and experiences.

It has been very important to enable Arnold Lodge patients to decide how they will relate to, and work with, the writer in residence. For example, patients sometimes arrange to see him, but change their minds the following week. It is always made clear that they are welcome to do this; and that decisions about whether to meet, and the nature of any work undertaken, depends on their choice.

Many patients have, understandably, needed to establish a level of trust before engaging in formal written work. For example, one group of patients initially invited the writer in residence to watch *Eastenders* with them. This then led to a discussion, on patients' terms, of the storyline and the plot; and an examination of how writers construct 'cliffhangers': eg. was Steve going to be sent down for accidentally killing his ex-girlfriend? The writer in residence has also established trust and confidence through participation in pool and other games. As patients are usually more skilled than the writer, they often take on the role of teacher, explaining, for example, the taking of shots. From such general discussions, some patients have started to talk spontaneously about their writing.

Throughout the residency, the writer in residence has been concerned to create situations and develop trust, in order that writers can find and use their own voice. An example is one individual who wished to write poems which were close to the text of the romantic poets. His enthusiasm for this type of poetry was acknowledged, but the writer in residence used this as a springboard for him to write about his own experiences in his own words. The writer in residence enabled another individual to describe his life experiences in his first language and to compose a recipe and write about his cultural and religious experiences.

Two individuals wished to create rap and hip-hop lyrics. The writer in residence enabled them to bring their own music into the session, write a lyric reflecting their own experience of prison life; and relate this to popular lyrics concerning struggles. He listened to their views about oppression in prison and psychiatric systems and enabled them to express this.

For many patients, finding their voice has meant enabling them to converse, write or read in their own language or preferred mode of communication, including music. One individual, who had not been in the UK very long, took the opportunity to voice concerns about racism, oppression and isolation within English society. After several angry outbursts, this led to the composition of two love songs, in collaboration with the writer in residence.

One patient initially expressed quite frankly her distrust of anyone, particularly a writer, and then decided to meet with the writer in residence each week to discuss various topics, initially her love of sixties and seventies pop music, and sometimes, complaints about psychiatric regimes. Often, the session resulted in the writing of pop lyrics, and significantly, accounts of happy memories such as bonfire night and Christmas.

Writing as a gift and patient ownership

Some patients have felt empowered from being enabled to make a gift of their writing to a loved one. This has included poems for girlfriends, boyfriends, partners and spouses; and in particular, poems written in condolence or as a gift to a relative who has died, or to another member of the patient's family. In several instances, writing has re-established communication with family members with whom patients had lost contact.

Patients' ownership of their writing is particularly important. Any work produced by patients is treated as confidential and is kept by them. The only exception to confidentiality would be if an individual mentioned an intention to harm self or others. This has never been mentioned in sessions, but if the topic arose, the individual would be told that, to ensure safety, this would be passed onto a registered nurse on his/her ward.

Creative versus therapeutic writing

Reference was made earlier to the need for clarity of the aims of the residency and the distinction between creative and therapeutic uses of writing. While it is necessary to be clear about this distinction in relation to aims, for some patients creative writing may lead to therapeutic gains in the broadest sense, as a by-product, rather than an intention of the sessions. Several individuals have commented on feeling positive about the work they have produced; and a few patients have used writing as a safe way to express anger or other feelings about the past.

Some patients have expressed surprise or excitement at producing work for the first time. One man was delighted and astonished at his first poem. Another individual, who had never tried creative writing previously, has composed at least one poem a week for over a year. He was pleased to have produced a word-processed collection of work for competition submission. Several patients have won Koestler Awards in an annual competition for people in secure hospitals and prisons. One individual has had several pieces accepted for publication.

Conclusion

Those of us who have experienced mental health problems are often perceived only as 'service users', with the added label of 'mentally disordered offender' (a term used routinely by professionals, but rarely questioned) if we are patients in secure facilities.

> *Mental health professionals and other social care workers, alongside non-experts, find it easier to focus on discrete elements in the individual's life: their 'illness', their service use. ... For many societies, the diagnosed-mentally ill as* **service user** *or* **consumer of mental health care** *appears to be easier to countenance than the diagnosed — mentally-ill as citizen or human being.*

(Barker *et al*, 1999, p. xv. emphasis in the original)

We would argue that admission to any mental health facility, including secure units, should enable not only individuals' assessment and the amelioration or resolution of particular problems, but their discovery of positive coping strategies, abilities, attributes and talents. Creative writing is one among many ways to enable this discovery, and for some individuals to 'find a voice'.

Key points

⌘ Creative writing can enable empowerment through providing people with a 'voice' to express their experiences and perspectives.

⌘ A writer-in-residency was established at Arnold Lodge medium secure unit, initially with funding from the Poetry Society's Poetry Places scheme. General principles to ensure the success of a writing residency in enabling empowerment are proposed, based on the authors' experience.

⌘ Writing residencies should always be in response to the expressed needs of clients, rather than imposed on them. The residency was established because of several patients' specific interests, and general dissatisfaction with leisure activities, expressed in a survey.

⌘ The success of a residency involves careful selection and the writer's welcome and introduction to the organisation. (S)he should be seen as a valued member of the service, who contributes a different, 'outsider' perspective. Induction, supervision, support and appropriate resources for the writer are essential.

⌘ At Arnold Lodge, careful planning and proposals, acceptable to powerful people in the organisation, and enlisting their support, were felt to be important. Participation of patients was limited at the planning stage to avoid disappointing their expectations, and to establish that managers and staff agreed with the project.

⌘ A distinction needs to be made between aims of writing as a creative leisure activity, and as a 'therapy'. However, the former may lead to broad therapeutic benefits, such as positive feelings about work produced.

⌘ Good communication is important, as is identification of, and application for, appropriate funding. Communication about the Arnold Lodge residency, with patients, managers, staff and funding bodies, is described.

⌘ Writers in residence need to be sensitive to the perspectives of clients, who should be free to choose the type and method of working with the writer. The establishment of trust and confidentiality is vital, as is the need for flexibility and accessibility. Ways of achieving these aims in the Arnold Lodge residency are described.

⌘ A wide variety of prose and poetry was produced by Arnold Lodge patients. Among many functions, the writing has helped patients communicate in their first language, give voice to their experiences and perspectives, produce poems as a gift and re-establish communication with families. Several patients have won awards, and one individual has had work published.

References

Adams D (1979) *The Hitch-Hiker's Guide to the Galaxy*. Pan Books Ltd, London

Barker P, Campbell P, Davidson B (1999) Preface. In: Barker P, Campbell P, Davidson B, eds. *From the Ashes of Experience. Reflection on Madness, Survival and Growth*. Whurr Publishers, London

Fisher D (1999) Hope, Humanity and Voice in Recovery from Mental Illness, quoting The Journal of the California Alliance for the Mentally Ill. In: Barker P, Camp bell P, Davidson B, eds. *From the Ashes of Experience. Reflection on Madness, Survival and Growth*. Whurr Publishers, London: chap 8

Kemshall H, Littlechild R (2000) Research Informing Practice. Some Concluding Remarks. In: Kemshall H, Littlechild R, eds. *User Involvement and Participation in Social Care*. Jessica Kingsley, London: chap 14

Lees N, Withington J (2001) Involving service users. In: Dale C, Thompson T, Woods P, eds. *Forensic Mental Health. Issues in Practice*. Baillière Tindall/Royal College of Nursing, Edinburgh, chap 11

Leicestershire Community Health Council and Arnold Lodge Education and Quality Department (1998) *Patient Satisfaction Survey* (1998). Unpublished Report

Leicestershire Community Health Council and Arnold Lodge Education and Quality Department (2000) *Patient Satisfaction Survey*. Unpublished Report

McArdle S, Byrt R (2001) Fiction, poetry and mental health: expressive and therapeutic uses of literature. *J Psychiatr Mental Health Nurs*

Sampson F (1999) *The Healing Word. A Practical Guide to Poetry and Personal Development Activities*. The Poetry Society, London

Ward D (2000) Totem not Token: Groupwork as a Vehicle for User Participation. In: Kemshall H, Littlechild R, eds. *User Involvement and Participation in Social Care*. Jessica Kingsley, London: chapter 3

21

Conclusions

James Dooher and Richard Byrt

This book will conclude with a summary based on the contributions to this book and other literature, including the benefits and problems of empowerment and participation and the factors which facilitate and hinder attempts, by individuals and organisations, to increase the extent to which service users and carers are empowered and have opportunities for participation.

The benefits and problems of empowerment and participation

Many benefits and problems of empowerment and participation have been described in the contributions to this book, its companion volume (*Empowerment and Participation: Power, influence and control in contemporary health care*), and in other literature. These are summarised in *Table 21.1*.

Table 21.1: Benefits and problems of empowerment and participation

Benefits	⇔	Problems
1. May result in increases in individual (psychological) empowerment, eg. raised self-efficacy, self-esteem, self-confidence, self-worth and pride in identity.	⇔	1. May lead to decreases in individual (psychological) empowerment, particularly if strategies to increase participation fail to take account of individuals' wishes to be involved and their specific aptitudes, self-beliefs and skills.
2. Has the potential to value the individual service user/carer and his/her views.	⇔	2. Service users/carers likely to feel devalued if their views are not taken seriously or acted on, or if there is tokenism or 'pseudo-participation'.
3. Service users/carers benefit from opportunities for their perspectives to be voiced and appreciated. This also enables professionals and managers to provide services which meet the expressed needs of service users/carers.	⇔	3. If there is a clash of perspective, professionals and managers may be especially likely to dictate the extent and nature of empowerment and participation.
4. Reported benefits from involvement in decision making and responsibility.	⇔	4. Individuals can be disempowered if there is a mismatch between their wish for empowerment/participation and the expectations of others.
5. Information, explanation and consultation may be valued by some service users/carers, whether or not their power is increased or participation at higher levels is involved. Some service users/carers do not want higher levels of participation.	⇔	5. According to some authors, true empowerment and participation cannot occur unless there are changes in the distribution of power. In the view of these authors: ⌘ Information, explanation and consultation in isolation do not constitute true participation.
6. Mutual giving and receiving of support in some participatory mechanisms, eg. self-help groups.	⇔	6. Not all individuals feel able, or wish to be involved in this way. The giving of support may be left to a few participants.
7. Participation of service users/carers, including the expression of their views and choices, helps to ensure that services meet their needs.	⇔	7. The views, choices and other participation of service users/carers may: a) conflict with other organisational goals and priorities; b) be difficult to take forward because of lack of resources.
8. In professional-client communication and relationships based on empowerment and participation models, there is greater emphasis on equality, a partnership approach, and respect for the expertise of the service user/carer.	⇔	8. Some service users/carers want a professional relationship and communication in which they play a passive role, with the professional as expert.

9. Service user/carer participation has contributed to improvements in services.	⇔	9. Such participation has often not resulted in improvements related to: a) issues of most importance to service users/carers; b) changes in wider society related to increased social inclusion and life opportunities.
10. The skills of service users and carers benefit both other people in similar circumstances, and in specific health services.	⇔	10. Service users and carers may consider that they lack requisite skills, or organisations may fail to recognise the skills they have. Resources may be needed to enable both service users/carers and professionals to gain skills in relation to empowerment and participation.
11. Many empowerment and participation approaches emphasise the rights of service users and carers.	⇔	11. Charters of Rights for service users and carers in health services in the UK are not legally enforceable, and may not be reflected in practice. The rights of some individuals may conflict with their responsibilities or the rights of other service users or carers, the public or professionals.
12. Empowerment and participation in community health projects is often found to increase social cohesion and decrease isolation.	⇔	12. Some people may not desire these goals. Other goals may be more important to them.
13. Empowerment and participation can lead to action, and successfully bring about change.	⇔	13. The extent of change often depends on resources and the decisions of people in positions of power.
14. Some service users and carers prefer representation by others. Other individuals, including professionals, may not be representative of their constituencies.	⇔	14. Service users and carers who actively participate are not representative of other service users and carers.

Factors facilitating and hindering empowerment and participation

The next part of this chapter summarises contributors' comments on factors which facilitate or hinder empowerment and participation. A large number of such factors have been identified by contributors to this book, its companion volume and other authors. These factors can be categorised under three headings:

1.   Clarity, or lack of clarity, in relation to conceptualisation, aims, goals, policies and strategies.

2. The motivation, commitment and abilities of different participants: people in positions of power, politicians, service users, informal carers, professionals and managers.
3. Resources, organisational and other structures, and specific methods used to facilitate or hinder empowerment and participation.

Conceptualisation

Byrt and Dooher (Dooher and Byrt, 2002, chapter 2) considered the importance of being aware of the meaning of empowerment and participation, and the complexity and multidimensional nature of these concepts, as applied in practice. It was argued here that the successful implementation of policies and strategies for more formal types of empowerment and participation is, in part, dependent on clarity about the nature of what is to be achieved, in relation to the degree, level and other dimensions of empowerment and participation. Ann Jackson and John Hyslop cite the comment of Glenister (1994) that, in various studies, '... theoretical frameworks for defining participation were largely inadequate...'. These contributors also quote Mullender and Ward (1991), who emphasise the importance of applying concepts of empowerment to practice. Although clarity of method for the successful implementation of empowerment or participation is urged in Byrt and Dooher (2002), this is not enough in itself. Tony Booth points out that in some local authorities, the methods for enabling communication and consultation may be clearly articulated, but 'remain largely unrealised', with no monitoring of implementation in practice: rhetoric rather than reality (*Chapter 5*).

Clarity of aims and goals is also seen by some authorities to be an essential precursor of increases in empowerment and participation (see Dooher and Byrt, 2002, chapter 1). This is emphasised in accounts of several projects in this book, including self-help groups, establishing a writer in residence, the SHAPE and CHOICES projects, and the Somerset Health Panels. However, Rowden (2002) points out that establishing participation in high secure hospitals can be difficult because of a conflict between '... the therapeutic goal... [and] prison-like values and associated culture in publications from officialdom...'. In response to this point, we suggest that it is essential to be clear about both the importance of empowerment and participation, compared with other goals; and whether these are separate from, or intrinsic to, other organisational goals. Related to this, is clarity about the limits of involvement. Penelope Campling (*Chapter 10*) refers to the imperative for professional accountability as limiting democracy in a therapeutic community, and the need to ensure that, for example, opportunities for residents to have freedom of expression do not result in racist comments being tolerated. Mahendra Solanki and Richard Byrt (*Chapter 20*) outline the importance of being clear about the extent of client and managerial power when facilitating the entry of a writer in residence into an organisation. Martin Carter and Nicky Pearson (*Chapter 15*) comment on the need for health service managers to be honest about limits to public influence on policy making, with the need for clarity about, '... having to work within certain constraints and restrictions...'.

Specific procedures and methods

Several contributors refer to specific procedures, policies and strategies to facilitate empowerment and participation. In relation to arts projects, Jackie Green and Keith Tones state that, '... the participatory models which worked best were 'well structured, well organised' (*Chapter 19*). Tony Booth comments on the need for flexibility in methods to facilitate participation, and other contributors outline specific policies or procedures: eg. in relation to public participation, the setting up of self-help groups and complaints. Khoosal (2002) states that, '... open consultation exercises with inbuilt planned monitoring and evaluation of developments will meet the needs of black and other minority ethnic groups...'. Several contributors outline the importance of meetings as a means to facilitate or hinder empowerment and participation. The setting up and running of meetings, as a means to facilitate or hinder empowerment and participation, is outlined by several contributors. The need to ensure accessibility and convenient times and venues for meetings (Khoosal, 2002) are also considered. A few contributors describe meetings which are intimidating and alienating to service users and carers, eg. in relation to complaints. Tony Booth describes the considerable difficulties which some social services clients have encountered in relation to meetings, and the practical steps which need to be taken to ensure that parents with, say, responsibilities to young children, are able to attend. He comments: '... Service users need to have a say about where meetings are held and how meetings are to be run...

service users are not given any say over who attends meetings...'. The anonymous contributor refers to an inflexible structure and protocol: '... feelings and emotions are... generally alien to planning meeting procedures... [There was] a "conform or be excluded" pressure...'.

Language is also mentioned by several contributors. Khoosal (2002) emphasises the need for freedom from jargon, and for interpreters and information in an individual's first language. The anonymous contributor remarks on the use of jargon '... hugely offensive to service users...'. Some contributors refer to the pre-dominance of particular professional discourses, resulting in specific service users' and carers' perspectives being ignored. Tony Booth comments on the need for professionals to '... take care to establish the preferred language of communication for both adults and childen...'. Many of the comments on meetings and language concern accessibility; and being 'user-friendly and equitable' (Khoosal, 2002).

It was suggested in Dooher and Byrt (2002) that consideration and use of the most appropriate methods was essential to the successful implementation of empowerment and participation. Several contributors describe particular methods, sometimes in detail (eg. in the setting up of specific projects and research studies). Accounts by contributors and other authors suggest that one factor of key importance is ensuring that methods are acceptable and accessible to service users and carers: that the means chosen to facilitate empowerment or participation are seen as appropriate, and chosen by them, and not imposed by people in positions of power. This has been outlined in relation to research projects on issues of concern to service users and carers (Kemshall and Littlechild, 2000; Priestley, 1999). Methods chosen need to be likely to achieve specific goals of increased empowerment or participation, and be suited to participants' needs, wish to participate, degree of self-efficacy, and cultural and other perspectives. Among many examples, contributors outline factors likely to ensure the success of self-help groups; projects for people of minority sexual orientations and identitites; pro-active use of the media; and arts projects, including those involving collaboration with other agencies. Methods of facilitating empowerment and participation are sometimes imaginative and use a variety of ideas and media. One example is 'forum theatre', which enabled participants to '... act out their ideas... Such participation enabled the audience to imagine change, act it out, and then reflect collectively on the change... this empowered the audience to take social action...' (Jackie Green and Keith Tones, *Chapter 19*, citing Paterson,1999).

The methods chosen depend, in part, on whether aims and goals encompass consumerist or democratic participation. Thus, some of the arts projects described were intended to enable democratic participation: to mobilise community action to bring about social change. This can be the purpose of some meetings, in which service users and carers make decisions related to participation; but other meetings may be used solely for people in power to announce decisions already made, or for a pretence at consultation. Alternatively, meetings can be used for consumerist participation, eg. for managers to ascertain service users' or carers' views or to listen to complaints and concerns. Problems can arise (as appears to have happened in the meetings described by the anonymous contributor), when there are differences in opinion about the aims of particular meetings, and concerning the extent of power and participation of service users and carers. Agreement about the aims of meetings (and of any other methods) appears to be important for the achievement of successful participation and empowerment.

Collaboration versus opposition

Some of the literature suggests that the most appropriate method, and the degree and level of participation aimed for, also depends, in part, on an accurate assessment of the goals and priorities of an organisation, and of the relative amounts of power of different participants. The mode of intervention, collaborative or oppositional, towards people in power depends partly on participants' position in, or in relation to, the organisation. There is evidence that individuals who are employed by, or receive funding from, an organisation (eg. a voluntary organisation receiving funding from a local or national statutory body) may find it harder to take a critical stance towards it, or oppose those in power within it, compared to independent opponents (Wood, 2000). This is one reason why the notion that nurses are in a position to advocate for service users has been criticised (Teasdale, 1998). If staff employed by an organisation are to keep their jobs, they may need to introduce ideas for empowerment or participation to managers in the first instance, before approaching service users. Such collaborative approaches may result in incremental approaches to participation, with the latter dictated on the terms of managers and professionals. Tony Booth argues that approaches which fail to challenge power or urge its redistribution, '... Merely [serve] to preserve the status quo in a new and more acceptable form...'. However, Keith Tones and Jackie Green refer to the value of coalitions in community projects, and the use of mediation: '... Compromise... between different and conflicting interests...'. More gains in (limited) participation, particularly of a consumerist nature, may be achieved in the long term if projects are agreed by people in positions of power (see *Chapter 20*). The alternative is to be either independent of, or an opponent within the system, as was described in Rowden (2002). Opposition within the system generally requires allies and/or a senior position in the organisation, and charismatic and other leadership qualities. Some managers and professionals have used their collaboration with voluntary organisations and other independent bodies to bring about changes, including increased service user participation, within statutory services (Byrt, 2001).

Tony Booth refers to the importance of monitoring and the sharing of good practice. Evaluating the extent to which empowerment and participation have increased, following the introduction of particular projects and methods, can help to establish which of the latter are effective with specific groups of service users and carers, and in relation to particular dimensions of empowerment and participation. This can then be applied to future attempts to empower individuals and enable their participation (Kemshall and Littlechild, 2000).

Successful participation and empowerment is likely to facilitate increased future gains in these areas. Jackie Green and Keith Tones, citing Putnam, 1995, comment on the boosts to psychological empowerment which can result from successful community participation. This makes it more likely that participants, '... will take up other causes. The vicious circle of learned helplessness can gradually be turned round into a virtuous circle of participation and empowerment...'. Equally, adverse experiences of supposedly participatory processes may deter individuals from future attempts to be involved, as has been the case with some people's efforts to use current health service complaints procedures.

Examples of facilitating, and failing to facilitate, consumerist participation, have been considered in Dooher and Byrt (2002), in relation to equality, information and explanation, voice, choice, control and autonomy, and accessibility, availability, redress (eg. through complaints systems) and rights and advocacy. These areas can be seen as important components of empowerment and participation, particularly consumerist participation. In addition, where these components exist (eg. in health services) they may also facilitate further development in empowerment and participation at different degrees and levels. Some contributors argue that provision of these areas in health services, and effective professional communication, in particular (see below) can enhance individual (psychological) empowerment. Contributors vary in their accounts of the extent that involvement in lower levels of participation, such as information and consultation, enabled psychological empowerment or participation at higher levels.

The next part of this chapter considers the influence of Government, service users and carers, professionals and managers on empowerment and participation.

The influence of central Government

Most of the contributors mention references to empowerment and participation in various central Government documents. Bob Sang (*Chapter 3*) points out that it is only in the past twenty years that public authorities have begun to address the issue of patient and public participation in health systems by identifying ways and means of engaging with lay people which supplemented traditional, formal duties to consult. In the last two decades, participation, and more recently, empowerment, have been mentioned in an increasing number of documents, many of which are referred to by contributors. These include legislation and various Department of Health papers, concerned, among other things, with service users' views, wishes, needs and rights. Examples mentioned by contributors include the Mental Health Act 1983, the Children Act 1989, the NHS and Community Care Act 1990, the Carers (Recognition and Services) Act 1995, the Disability Discrimination Act 1995 and the Human Rights Act 1998; as well as Department of Health papers, such as National Service Frameworks and *Clinical Governance: Quality in the New NHS*. Few contributors mention *Patient and Public Involvement in the NHS* (DoH, 1999), but several contributors refer to the *NHS Plan* (NHS Executive, 2000), in which service user and carer participation is particularly stressed:

> ... *For the first time, patients will have a real say in the NHS. They will have new powers and more influence over the way the NHS works...*
>
> (NHS Executive, 2000, quoted in Gillam, 2001, p. 27)

The meeting of some needs and rights of certain service users and carers is enshrined in legislation and Department of Health documents, and some contributors give positive examples of this in practice, eg. in relation to primary care and National Institute for Clinical Excellence requirements on service users' views. The anonymous contributor (*Chapter 8*) comments that his suggestions concerning language in local reports, 'met with some success, as Government guidelines... included such provision...'. Roberta Wetherell-Graley outlines her own influence, as a former service user, on UK and European government policy. Keith Tones and Jackie Green (2002) comment on the World Health Organization's commitment to empowerment, eg. through the establishment of 'active participating communities'.

However, some other contributors question the extent to which legislation and Government policy on service users' and carers' views and participation works in practice. The anonymous contributor comments: '... I achieved little, if anything, for local service users by my involvement. I had, however, met Government requirements for "user involvement" at a strategic level...'. Breeze (2002) comments, in relation to the Disability Discrimination Act 1995, that there is a '... long way to go before people with mental health problems and social disability achieve equality...'. This point has also been made with reference to individuals with physical disabilities (Casserley, 2000; Priestley, 1999). Nessa McHugh (*Chapter 4*) argues that *Changing Childbirth* has had little influence on mothers' participation in decisions concerning childbirth; and Sue Evans and Richard Byrt report research suggesting widespread dissatisfaction with complaints procedures, despite the arrangements in *Acting on Complaints* (DoH, 1995). Many carers are said to be unaware of their rights under the Carers (Recognition and Services) Act (Rogers, 2000). Nessa McHugh and Tony Booth point out that professionals are sometimes unaware of national and local patients'/clients' charters. Furthermore, legislation and other Government documents related to service users' and carers' views and rights may be contradicted by other legislation. For example, increased powers to enforce treatment in the community (under the proposed new Mental Health Act for England and Wales) limit mental health clients' participation in their care (Beresford and Croft, 2001). Jane Gregory refers to discriminatory attitudes towards gay men and lesbians implicit in the Local Government Act, 1988 (yet to be repealed at the time of writing). Lawrence Whyte and Gerry Carton comment on Government directives which place '... re-emphasis upon the primacy of the protection of the public...', at the expense of the rights and needs of patients in high secure hospitals. Other contributors criticise free market legislation in the 1980s and 1990s. Breeze (2002) points out that despite its stated intentions, this failed to offer choice in the NHS.

The influence of service users and carers

This book includes several examples of empowerment and participation initiated by service users and carers themselves. *Chapter 3* considered the clear identification of 'service users' as important to the success of strategies to increase empowerment and participation. Some health services can be seen as having a wide range of 'service users', in the sense of stakeholders or people with an interest in the service. These may include members of the public, the local media, voluntary organisations, politicians and the Department of Health (Byrt, 2001). Managers may decide that the interests of these groups, as well as those of clients/patients and carers need to be met. The possible conflict of interest between high secure hospital patients and members of the public is identified by several contributors in this volume and in Dooher and Byrt (2002). In addition, service users and carers may also have different needs. Jenny Fisher (*Chapter 12*) and Tony Booth (*Chapter 5*) indicate this, respectively, in relation to people with schizophrenia and their carers, and children and their parents. A recognition of such possible differences appears to be important in developing strategies for participation.

Another important influence is the extent to which individual clients/patients and their carers desire empowerment and participation. In *Chapter 1* it was concluded that there is a need for professionals to assess this where possible, so that there is a match between the service user's/carer's wish to participate, and the actual opportunities to do so. There is a paradox, in that individuals can be encouraged, or even coerced, into being empowered or participating when they do not want this!

Individual motivation can be important, not only in relation to the participation of an individual service user or carer, but in enabling the empowerment and participation of other people in similar circumstances (Byrt, 1994). This motivation is implicit in the accounts by service users and carers in this book. In addition, several contributors consider the empowerment and participation of individuals or of service users or carers in general.

Representativeness and motivation to participate

In the literature, representativeness is frequently seen as a problem, with participants in various areas often said to be atypical of the groups which they purport to represent, and sometimes, inhibiting the participation of other individuals. A related problem is that in service user — or carer — run initiatives, most participants may not wish to take an active part. This may result in one or two individuals being left with most of the work of the organisation: a problem described by Andrew Wetherell in relation to self-help groups (*Chapter 17*) and by voluntary organisation participants in the research by Byrt (1994). Andrew comments on:

> *... how easy it can be for a highly motivated and enthusiastic person to get 'burnt-out' whilst running a self-help group... This... needs to be avoided as far as possible, with the various tasks within the group being shared. This not only leads to reduced pressures on the one or two naturally active individuals, but it also assists all participants to have... ownership of the group... .*

Involving many members of a local community is one way of possibly sharing the responsibility for participation, as in projects described by Jackie Green and Keith Tones (*Chapter 19*), and Larry Butler (2002). In one event, a Lantern Festival, '... everyone's contribution mattered... People... passed on [their] skills to others. The contacts and networks built up then provided an ongoing source of more general information and support...'.

Possible reasons for lack of participation include lack of time, as is said to be the case in relation to citizens' active political participation (Reznick, 1997). It is suggested that professionals need to be aware of time constraints on service users and carers when considering strategies for participation. Cost can be another factor, and may inhibit the participation of service users with limited income. Tony Booth comments that, to ensure this, help may need to be given with '... costs of childcare...' , with times for meetings matching the commitments of parents. Another aspect of cost is energy. Evans and Byrt (2002) review literature on the huge amount of energy and persistence needed to pursue complaints, at times when complainants are ill, bereaved or concerned about the care of a loved one. Energy is also needed by respondents in research which is service user or carer focused: a point which should always be remembered by researchers

(Kemshall and Littlechild, 2000). There may also be other costs to respondents, such as possible distress or pain related to the research topic (Byrt and Rees, 1999; Littlechild and Glasby, 2000). However, Cutcliffe (2002) reports that bereaved respondents in his study welcomed opportunities to give their views. His findings suggest that, in general, service users and carers should themselves be able to make decisions about participation in research studies, and that some ethics committees may be unnecessarily paternalistic in relation to this area.

Psychological empowerment, skills and abilities

Tones and Green (2002) suggest that the degree of individual (psychological) empowerment is also crucial in determining individuals' wish to participate, including taking action for community empowerment. Factors of importance include the degree of self-efficacy, self-esteem and self-confidence. The extent to which service users and carers possess (and perhaps, think they possess) relevant skills, abilities and talents is relevant to psychological empowerment. '... The development of skills... will contribute to self-efficacy beliefs, confidence and a sense of control... enhancement of self-esteem... if those involved feel that they are achieving worthwhile goals, then the meaningfulness of their involvement will lead to an enhanced sense of coherence...' (*Chapter 19*, citing Antonovsky, 1984). Several other contributors also refer to the importance of service users' skills: the development of those they possess, and acquiring new aptitudes and abilities. Wendy Ifill describes benefits from her development of various skills (*Chapter 11*). Whyte and Carton (2002) comment on the importance of, '... recognising the client's strengths, capabilities, potential and talents...'. In relation to expressive writing, Solanki and Byrt write: '... Several individuals have commented on feeling positive at producing work for the first time. One man was delighted and astonished at his first poem...'.

The skills, abilities and talents of service users and carers can result in participation at various degrees and levels, and enable them to contribute positively to individual care and treatment and service development. The possible need to identify specific skills in relation to particular types of participation is considered below .

Another factor related to service user and carer empowerment and participation concerns the individual's meeting other people in similar circumstances. A number of contributors have indicated the resultant lessening of isolation. '...[B]y meeting other people who felt the same as me, I really felt a sense of belonging...', writes Kevin (*p. 126*). For individuals who face discrimination, meeting others in similar circumstances may result in identification with them, a raising of consciousness and a pride in one's identity. These increases in psychological empowerment may enable individuals to help other people facing the same difficulties, in relation to social attitudes and wider discrimination and/or the practicalities of living with a particular illness. Advocacy, self-help groups and campaigning may help to achieve this, either in separatist groups of people with similar experiences, or in partnership with other people (Chamberlin, 1988).

The role of professionals

The accounts by contributors and other authors suggest that the role of professionals is also crucial to the success of some types of empowerment and participation. Several contributors mention the importance of aspects of professional–service user/carer communication and relationships. Topics described as affecting empowerment or participation, and considered in Dooher and Byrt (2002), include valuing individuals and their views and perspectives; active listening; self-awareness; awareness of negative attitudes (within oneself and in wider society) towards particular groups of people; and enabling the 'voice' of service users and carers. These items can be seen both as components of empowerment and as its 'facilitators'; and include the 'components of an effective empowering encounter' and Onyett's guidelines for engagement (Whyte and Carton, 2002) (see, also, Rogers, 1978, for aspects of interpersonal relationships said to facilitate empowerment). It has been argued that the giving of information and explanation is the lowest degree of participation (Byrt and Dooher, 2002). In contrast, information has also been viewed as 'the lower end' of a '... continuum [of "user involvement", with] participation and empowerment at the higher end...' (Brooks, 2001, citing Poulton, 1999).

The professional–service user/carer relationship is also seen by many contributors to be an important facilitating (or hindering) factor. In *Chapter 1*, it was pointed out that service users and carers vary in their desire for participatory relationships. It is often assumed that the latter are always a good thing. However, some individuals may prefer a professional to take control, especially during a crisis or an episode of acute illness:

> ... *The evidence that patients want to share decision making with doctors is... equivocal, and more research is needed to elucidate which patients, in which circumstances, want and will benefit from shared decision making...*

(Florin and Coulter, 2001, p. 44)

Models of professional–service user/carer relationship

The nature of the professional–service user/carer relationship, and the theoretical model informing it, is of particular relevance to the facilitation of empowerment and participation. Mike Saks (2002) traces the development of medical dominance in healthcare decision making, and concludes: '... orthodox biomedicine... has proved a major challenge to the power and empowerment of the consumer...'. A number of other contributors comment with concern on the power of professionals, particularly doctors, with Ray Rowden (2002) and Bob Sang (*Chapter 3*) referring to instances of ill treatment and neglect, particularly by nursing staff. The failure of some managers and professionals to acknowledge mistakes or take complaints seriously is reviewed in the chapter on this topic. In relation to social work, Tony Booth comments: '... contemporary practice is dominated by a "professionals know best" mentality. Although written agreements between workers and service users are becoming more common, whether they are used or not is generally the decision of practitioners who also determine most of the content... The position is made worse by the fact that some theoretical models informing social work practice actually militate against user participation in decision making...'. Judy Reece and Carrie White (2002) comment on ways in which mental health nurses' disempowering practices may be influenced by socialisation during their training and their own disempowerment. Strong socialising influences may result in the ostracisation of staff who advocate rights of patients, or try to increase the latter's empowerment or participation.

Several contributors outline empowering professional – service user/carer relationships which facilitated empowerment and participation, eg. in a therapeutic community (*Chapter 10*), in the care of a relative (*Chapter 13*) and in a variety of services. This area is examined, for example, in relation to avoidance of abusive practices in psychiatry (Khoosal, 2002); a ward philosophy to facilitate service user and carer participation; and creative writing. Nicky Pearson and Martin Carter (*Chapter 15*) conclude that partnerships between professionals and service users are now more frequent. '... Patients can now expect to be more involved in all aspects of the service...'. However, Florin and Coulter (2001) conclude: '... Despite the fact that it is possible to distinguish a historical trend towards patient-centred medicine, we do not really know how prevalent it is' (p. 46).

Related to professional–client relationships are attitudes towards service users and carers. Both empowering and disempowering attitudes (including downright discrimination) are described in this book. These attitudes, particularly those towards groups who face discrimination, may mirror those in wider society. (For an interesting, and very worrying, example of how this can affect nurse care planning, see Mercer *et al*, 1999.) As was pointed out by Byrt and Dooher (2002), this wider discrimination can often seriously militate against active participation in life opportunities, and make it impossible to achieve the fourth (social inclusion) dimension of empowerment. Sayce (2000) has commented that social exclusion towards certain groups of people, eg. individuals with mental illness is often taken for granted, widely accepted and seen as acceptable. Rowden (2002) describes how, sadly, such attitudes have been perpetuated in some mental 'health' hospitals. Paul Fitzgerald (*Chapter 7*) comments that there is, '... little acknowledgement of wider social discrimination by professionals...' in relation to people of minority sexual orientations and identities, and describes the development of a service to affirm the identity of these individuals and increase their self-esteem.

Power sharing

The extent to which professionals and managers are prepared to share power is also seen by some contributors to be important to certain types of participation and empowerment. This has sometimes depended on the perceived status of the patient and the extent to which service users'/carers' opposing views are tolerated. Nicky Pearson and Martin Carter (*Chapter 15*) state that managers should be, '... prepared to hear the unexpected and embrace it...'. Professional, legal and managerial accountability can limit professionals' attempts to increase empowerment and participation (Dimond, 2002). (An example concerns some midwives who enabled a mother to have a waterbirth at home, as she wished, but in doing so, found that their managers held them to account since trust policy did not cover waterbirths: Dimond, 1996.)

Some contributors refer to specific philosophies and models of care as empowering or disempowering, particularly biotechnical approaches in medicine; with concomitant failure to address psychological, social and spiritual factors and/or to affirm the individual and/or his/her identity often being mentioned. Judy Reece and Carrie White (2002), for example, mention '... heavy reliance on the medical model with women with borderline personality disorder...'. The anonymous contributor comments that, '... all the non-user representatives were major stakeholders in preserving the medical model...'. Service user control is said to rely heavily on the decisions of people in power. Part of power is reflected in discourse, and a number of contributors consider this in relation to the failure of many professionals to acknowledge the perspectives of mental health service users (*Chapter 2*); women using childbirth services (*Chapter 4*); and lesbians, gay men and individuals who are transgendered (*Chapter 6* and *7*). Poor standards of nursing or other care can also be experienced as disempowering. Related to both power and perspectives is assessment of need and decisions about treatment, with some professionals considering that their opinions in relation to this are the only 'expert' ones. According to Jayne Breeze (2002), for 'voice' to lead to empowerment, service users' requests for changes should be: '... taken on board by community mental health nurses... Nurses do not always hear [service users'] needs, choices and aspirations... maybe because they focus upon their own assessment of need and priority of goals...'.

The empowering or disempowering organisation

Some aspects of organisations, including structures, have been considered earlier in this chapter. This section considers organisational systems, and the extent to which they facilitate or hinder empowerment and participation. Several contributors describe damaging and abusive organisational cultures, particularly in secure and other mental health services. ('Organisational culture' is, '...a pervasive way of life or set of norms... deep-set beliefs about the way work should be organised, the way authority should be exercised, people rewarded, people controlled...' [Handy, 1993, quoted in Byrt, 2001, p. 78].)

The failure to treat 'service users' as individuals, the bad treatment and neglect in some organisations described in this book; and the discrimination described by other contributors, in relation to other services, can be seen as both a component of disempowerment and a factor which militates against the development of empowerment and participation. In the words of Bob Sang: '... All talk of patient involvement... is meaningless while we fail to address these issues of power and psychological damage in our health systems...'. In contrast, a few contributors describe organisations with cultures and environments which enabled empowerment and participation. Keith Tones and Jackie Green (2002) outline the key components of the World Health Organization's 'health promoting hospitals' (including requirements for patient and staff empowerment).

Resources

The editors suggest that an organisation's commitment to empowerment and participation is likely to be reflected in the amount of resources it allocates for their development. These are mentioned by several contributors. In relation to projects to increase participation and empowerment, Martin Carter and Nicky Pearson advise: '... Be realistic about the time and resources needed — including the level of expertise...'.

One resource is the appointment of a manager or staff member to take a lead in developing appropriate strategies and projects. Khoosal (2002) states that: '... Staff responsible for implementation need to be identified and a clear timetable for action ... made available...'; while Tony Booth refers to problems of implementation if there is no '... indication of who will take responsibility...'. Jackie Green and Keith Tones comment on the '... commitment, vision and enthusiasm of key individuals in setting up "Arts for health" projects...'.

The need for adequate training is stressed by several contributors, particularly for staff, and to ensure service user empowerment and 'cultural sensitivity' (Khoosal, 2002). Whyte and Carton (2002) describe the 'intellectual isolation' of certain disempowering institutions, with their lack of '... professional stimulus, training and education opportunities...'. Staff training, in relation to complaints is outlined by Evans and Byrt (2002). The importance of service user and carer training to ensure that participatory and empowerment processes work (*Chapter 5*); and enabling service users to acquire skills, '... and resources for self-expression' (*Chapter 19*) are also emphasised.

What factors need to be considered to increase service user and carer participation effectively?

This book will conclude with a consideration of factors which need to be considered in the implementation of strategies to increase formal, planned, as opposed to informal, empowerment and participation. This distinction is important, and is based on research by Byrt (1994: Byrt and Dooher, 2002) who found that participation in some voluntary organisations for mental health was spontaneous and unplanned, with no clear distinction between so-called 'service users' and other participants. Members enjoyed being together and taking part in activities in an *ad hoc* way and with a free spirit.

Most contributors to this book have described **planned** participation and empowerment. *Table 21.2 s*ummarises factors (many outlined in this book) which the editors propose need to be considered in relation to this more formal increase in involvement and power. However, we suggest (and this is indicated by some contributors) that it is necessary to be aware of some people's needs to participate in spontaneous ways, unfettered by policies and strategies. In any case, the latter need to be changing and dynamic, rather than rigid. Inflexible ideas about the nature of empowerment and participation, or how it should be facilitated, would themselves be likely to be a hindrance.

Table 21.2: Factors which need to be considered in facilitating formal empowerment and participation

A. Clear concepts, aims, goals, policies and stategies

1.	Clear conceptualisation. A clear idea of what 'empowerment' and 'participation' mean in relation to the service; and bearing in mind specific components, dimensions and models of empowerment and participation, including the degree and level to be achieved.
2.	Clarity of aims and goals of empowerment and participation.
3.	Specific strategies, and where appropriate, policies to achieve these aims and goals. Specific targets and dates to achieve them, where appropriate.
4.	Clarity about whether employment/participation is an **extrinsic** goal, separate from other organisational goals; or **intrinsic** to some or all of these goals.
5.	If empowerment/participation is extrinsic, clarity about its relative importance compared with other goals; and the extent that it complements or conflicts with them.
6.	Awareness of the mode of operation: eg. collaboration with, or opposition to, people in power; separatist or in partnership with other groups.
7.	Inclusion of empowerment/participation in the organisation's philosophy and mission statement, where appropriate.
8.	Decisions about the limits of empowerment and participation.

B. Service users, carers and organisational participants with power

1.	Clarity about which individuals constitute 'service users' and 'carers' (eg. do 'service users' include members of the public?)
2.	Awareness of similarities and differences between views of service users and carers, and different types of service user.
3.	Clarity about which organisational participants are to be active participants/empowered.
4.	Honest identification of the people in the organisation who are power holders; and the extent that they are prepared to share or devolve power.
5.	Awareness of the motivation and resources, including time, possessed by service users, carers and other participants, in relation to different types, levels and degrees of participation, and dimensions of empowerment, including care and the involvement of other service users/ carers.
6.	Awareness of, and provision of resources, as necessary, in relation to the nature and extent of: ⌘ particular skills of service users and carers ⌘ their psychological (individual) empowerment ⌘ opportunities to meet with others in similar circumstances, and for raising of consciousness and positive self-image.

C. Professionals, managers and Government departments

1.	Identification of particular individuals with responsibility for increasing empowerment/ participation.
2.	Professional/managerial communication and attitudes, involving: • self-awareness and reflection on practice • valuing service users/carers and their views and perspectives • positive, non-discriminatory attitudes and affirmation of identity, particularly of individuals stigmatised in wider society • active listening • enabling the voice of service users and carers • taking individuals, and their complaints and concerns seriously • opportunities for information and consultation.
3.	Accurate assessment of individual service users'/carers': • wish to participate and be empowered. Ensuring a match between desired participation and the amount of participation enabled by the professional/ manager • desire to challenge existing power holders and increase service user/carer power. Enabling service users/carers achieve the desired amounts of power.

4.	Identification of the extent that professionals/managers are prepared to: • share power and control • tolerate opposition and conflict.
5.	The type and nature of managerial and professional leadership.
6.	Particular philosophies and models of care and treatment, and their effect on professional-service/user relationships.
7.	Professional, legal, ethical and employment/managerial accountability, and its effect on empowerment/participation.
8.	Specific DoH and other central and local Government policies and strategies, their effects on empowerment/participation; and the extent that they are easy to implement in practice.
9.	Identification, and provision of, appropriate staff education, support and clinical supervision.
10.	Awareness of issues of language, discourse and meeting structure, and their effects on empowerment/participation. Provision of accessible, clear communication and meetings.

D. Specific areas

1.	Awareness of the specific components of empowerment/participation to be increased.
2.	Efforts to ensure social inclusion and life opportunities.
3.	Identification of anticipated and actual benefits and problems of empowerment and participation.
4.	Awareness and choice of the most appropriate method to increase empowerment/participation.
5.	Identification of specific resources needed, including funding and appropriate venues.
6.	Evaluation and monitoring of initiatives (including research) with particular reference to service users'/carers' experiences, benefits and problems, and facilitating and hindering factors.
7.	Making information available, both on good practice and on projects which were unsuccessful, with analysis of factors involved in facilitating and hindering empowerment/participation.
8.	Awareness of aspects of organisational culture which constrain, and provision of cultures which facilitate empowerment/participation.
9.	Awareness of the stages of projects at which carers/service users can be involved.

Conclusion

We hope that this book will add to the debate about empowerment and participation and their practical application in healthcare practice. During our work compiling this and its companion book (Dooher and Byrt, 2002) we have become increasingly aware of the vast amount of material that deserves inclusion. We look forward to writing further on this topic, and are interested in hearing from anyone who feels they have something to contribute. We are aware of gaps in our own understanding, and of areas of health care which are not covered. We appreciate the many contributions, and feel confident that these will add positively to the literature. We would like to conclude by thanking all the authors and readers of this book and its companion volume, for accompanying us in our journey to discover the meaning and practical application of empowerment and participation in health care.

James Dooher and Richard Byrt

References

Antonovsky A (1984) The sense of coherence as a determinant of health. In: Matarazzo JD *et al*, eds. *Behavioural Health*. John Wiley, New York

Beresford P, Croft S (2001) Mental health policy: a suitable case for treatment. In: Newnes C, Holmes G, Dunn C, eds. *This is Madness Too. Critical perspectives on mental health services*. PCCS Books, Ross on Wye: chapter 2

Breeze J (2002) User participation and empowerment in community mental health nursing practice. In: Dooher J, Byrt R, eds (2002a) *op cit*: chapter 6

Brooks F (2001) Why user involvement in primary health care? In: Gillam S, Brooks F, eds. *New Beginnings: Towards patient and public involvement in primary health care*. King's Fund/University of Luton, London: chapter 1

Butler L (2002) Empowerment and participation: the arts in health care. In Dooher J, Byrt R, eds (2002a) *op cit*: chapter 14

Byrt R (1994) *Consumer Involvement in a Voluntary Organisation for Mental Health*. Unpublished PhD Thesis, Loughborough University

Byrt R (2001) Power influence and control in practice development. In: Clark A, Dooher J, Fowler J, eds. *Handbook of Practice Development*. Quay Books Division, Mark Allen Publishing Limited, Salisbury

Byrt R, Dooher J (2002) Empowerment and Participation: Definitions, meanings and models. In: Dooher J, Byrt, eds. (2002a) *op cit*: chapter 2

Byrt R, Rees J (1999) Patients' perspectives of self-harm in a medium secure unit. *Mental Health Practice* 3(3): 30–4

Casserley C (2000) The Disability Discrimination Act: An overview. In: Cooper J, ed. *Law, Rights and Disability*. Jessica Kingsley Publishers, London: chapter 6

Chamberlin J (1988) *On Our Own. Patient Controlled Alternatives to the Mental Health System*. MIND Publications, London

Cutcliffe JR (2002) Ethics committees, vulnerable groups and paternalism: the case for considering the beliefs of participating in qualitative research interviews. In: Dooher J, Byrt R, eds (2002a) *op cit*: 13

Department of Health (1999) *Patient and Public Participation in the NHS*. Cited in: Gillam S (2001) *op cit*

Department of Health (1995) *Acting on Complaints. The Government's Revised Policy and Proposals for a New NHS Complaints Procedure in England*. March, 1995. EL (95) 37

Department of Health (1999) *The Government's Objectives for Children's Social Services*. HMSO, London

Department of Health (1995) The Carers' Recognition & Service Act

Dimond B (2002) *Legal Aspects of Nursing*. 3rd edn. Mosby, London

Dimond B (1996) *The Legal Aspects of Midwifery*. Books for Midwives Press, London

Disability Discrimination Act (1995) HMSO, London

Dooher J, Byrt R, eds (2002a) *Empowerment and Participation: Power, influence and control in contemporary health care*. Volume one. Quay Books, Mark Allen Publishing Limited, Salisbury

Dooher J, Byrt R (2002) Primary care. In: Dooher J, Byrt R, eds (2002a) *op cit*: chapter 4

Evans S, Byrt R (2002) The power to complain. In Dooher J, Byrt R, eds (2002a) *op cit*: chapter 15

Florin D, Coulter A (2001) Partnership in the primary care consultation. In: Gillam S, Brooks F *New Beginnings. Towards Patient and Public Involvement in Primary Health Care*. King's Fund/University of Luton, London: chapter 4

Gillam S (2001) Primary care: evolving policy. In: Gillam S, Brooks F *New Beginnings. Towards Patient and Public Involvement in Primary Health Care*. King's Fund/University of Luton, London: chapter 2

Glenister D (1994) Patient participation in psychiatric services: A literature review and proposal for a research strategy. *J Adv Nurs* **19**: 802–11

Handy C (1993) *Understanding Organisations*. 4th edn. Penguin Books, Harmondsworth

Human Rights Act (1998) HMSO, London

Kemshall H, Littlechild R (2000) Participation and involvement. In: Kemshall H, Littlechild R, eds. *User Involvement and Participation in Social Care*. Jessica Kingsley Publishers, London

Khoosal D (2002) Psychiatry and power. In: Dooher J, Byrt R, eds (2002a) *op cit*: chapter 10

Mercer D, Mason T, Richman J (1999) Good and evil in the crusade of care. *J Psychosoc Nurs and Ment Health Services* **37**(9): 13–17

Mullender A, Ward D (1985) Towards an alternative model of social groupwork. *Br J Social Work* **15**: 155–72

Poulton B (1999) User involvement in identifying health needs and shaping and evaluating services: is it being realised? *J Adv Nurs* **30**(6): 1289–96

Priestley M (1999) *Disability Politics and Community Care*. Jessica Kingsley Publishers, London

Read J, Wallcroft J (1992) *Guidelines for Empowering Users of Mental Health Services*. Confederation of Health Service Employees/MIND: London

Reece J, White C (2002) Women's empowerment — myth or reality. In: Dooher J, Byrt R, eds (2002a) *op cit*: chapter 7

Reznick P (1997) *Twenty-first Century Democracy*. McGill-Queen's University Press, Montreal

Rogers C (1978) *Carl Rogers on Personal Power. Inner Strength and Its Revolutionary Impact*. Constable, London

Rogers C (2000) Breaking the ice: developing strategies for collaborative working with carers of older people with mental health problems. In: Kemshall H, Littlechild J (2000) *op cit*: chapter 7

Rowden R (2002) Empowerment in forensic mental health: the challenge to leaders. In: Dooher J, Byrt R, eds (2002a) *op cit*: chapter 11

Saks M (2002) Empowerment, participation and the rise of orthodox biomedicine. In: Dooher J, Byrt R, eds (2002a) *op cit*: chapter 3

Sayce L (2000) *From Psychiatric Patient to Citizen. Overcoming Discrimination and Social Exclusion*. Macmillan, Basingstoke

Teasdale K (1998) *Advocacy in Health Care*. Blackwell Science, Oxford

Tones K, Green J (2002) The empowerment imperative in health promotion. In: Dooher J, Byrt R, eds(2002a) *op cit*: chapter 5

Whyte L, Carton G (2002) Creating and maintaining strategies for empowering clients within high secure hospital settings. In: Dooher J, Byrt R, eds (2002a) *op cit*: chapter 12

Wood B (2000) *Patient Power? The Politics of Patients' Associations in Britain and America*. Open University Press, Buckinghamshire

Index

A

abuse   22, 128, 154
~ child   154
~ family   106
~ in hospitals   52
~ sexual   109
~ verbal   8
~ personal boundaries   154
access to information   88
accessibility   55, 258, 263, 266
~ of health service documents   130
accident and emergency   173
accountability   54, 274
~ professional   148, 157
~ to public   214
Acting on Complaints   268
action   239
acute admission wards   149
advocacy   58, 95, 266, 272
~ carers   175, 178
~ nurses   265
~ service users   175
~ groups   7
ageism   138, 140, 205
aggression   166
AIDS   212
~ individuals living with   12, 209
~ patient activists   23
alcohol   154
Alcoholics Anonymous   205, 206
alienation   67, 106, 263
~ from health care   108
Alma Ata conference   231
Alton Towers   222
~ 'horror stories', reasons for   221
antibiotics   234
antidepressants   231

antipsychiatry   36
anti-stigma   220
anxiety   242
~ experience of   203
~ individuals with   208
approachability   177
army psychiatric services   146
Arnold Lodge   248
aromatherapy   160
art
~ as therapy   230
~ in health promotion   230
artist in residence   233
arts, the
~ benefits of   246
~ communication   230, 241
~ empowerment   230–231, 233, 235, 237, 239, 241, 243, 245, 247
~ feelings   230, 245
~ health promotion   245
~ in general practices   245
~ political statements   230, 245
~ quality of work   244, 246
~ satisfaction   236
~ space for   244
~ therapies   245
arts activities   248–249
arts for health projects   276
~ development of   246
~ evaluation of   242
arts in health   244
~ benefit of   244
~ cost-effectiveness of   244
~ organisations   244
arts projects   236, 263–265
~ feelings   235
~ schools   245
Ashworth Hospital   214– 215, 217, 219–220, 222–225, 227
~ 'horror stories'   221, 228

Health Development Agency (HDA) 242
Health Education Authority (HEA) 242, 244, 246
health improvement plans 232
health panels 187–188, 262
health promoting hospitals 276
health promotion 27, 230, 232, 244–245
health service 29
Health Service Ombudsman 173, 175
healthcare needs 110
health-related learning 234
healthy living centres 244
hearing
~ difficulties with 173
Henderson Hospital 147
heterosexism 101–102, 110–111, 113–114
heterosexual values 122
hierarchies 135
HIV 120, 212
~ individuals with 209
~ literature 111
~ testing 9
holism 169
holistic approach 121
homeostasis 155
homophily 235
homophobia 108, 110, 125
~ internalised 104–105, 115
homosexuality 125
honesty 175
horror stories 228
horticultural projects 174
Hospital Advisory Service 17
hospitals
~ conflict in goals 262
~ long-stay 17, 5153
~ secure 215, 225
hostage taking incident 220, 224
Human Rights Act 1998 267
humanities
~ and ethics 244

I

identity
~ and disability 8
~ minority sexual groups 274
~ older people 176
~ pride in 260, 272
ill health
~ experience of 235
~ writing about 235
ill treatment 273
illness
~ carcinomas 23
~ effect on participation 26
~ experience of 232
~ influence on participation 21
immunisation parties 233, 245
inclusion 48, 170
~ of lesbian/gay partners 109
individualism 147, 156
inequality 103, 139, 230–231, 245
influence
~ public 263
informal carers 196
information 13, 20, 24–28, 30, 173, 175, 178, 237, 239, 252, 266, 272
~ freedom of 213
~ in first language 264
~ journalists 228
~ lack of 175
~ media 213
Institute of Medical Humanities 231
institutionalisation 147
institutions 53
~ isolation 276
internal market 241
International Classification of Impairment, Disability and Handicap 7
Internet 72, 112
interpreters 264
involvement 48, 243
Irish people 128–129
isolation 108, 236–238, 246, 272